HEALTHY, SPEEDY, FREE! [5 BOOKS IN 1]

Improve Your Physical Condition with the Best
Therapeutic Movements and Lectin-Free Recipes to
Improve Circulation and Oxygenation of the Body

By

Lil Ron

Table of Contents

7-MINUTE WORKOUT FOR SENIORS

THE 15-DAY MEN'S HEALTH BOOK OF 15-MINUTE WORKOUTS

THE 15-DAY WOMEN'S HEALTH BOOK OF 15-MINUTE WORKOUTS

HYPNOSIS FOR WEIGHT LOSS

THE EASY LECTIN FREE COOKBOOK

7-Minute Workout for Seniors

By

Lil Ron

Table of Contents

Introduction

7-Minute Workout for Seniors is a fitness book that specifically focuses on the benefits of exercise for seniors. The idea of this book is to provide information and inspiration to ensure that seniors can continue to live active, healthy lifestyles in old age. This book provides both a workout regime as well as advice on how to prepare for it. Because this book focuses on older individuals, it also includes some useful information about growing old, reminding readers that aging need not mean the end of physical activity and comfort with one's body.

This book has been written with the intention that it can be used by anyone, regardless of their educational background. It includes information on the importance of regular exercise for a healthy lifestyle and details of various exercises that can be carried out without any special equipment. These exercises are particularly geared towards individuals who may not have much strength or energy but with practice, can become more comfortable with their bodies and begin to move more independently. This book has been well-received by users because it does not require any sort of specific pre-existing condition in order to make use of its contents. It does not focus on fitness in terms of weight loss but rather, as a means to improve quality of life for older individuals. It has also been praised for its multiple useful tips which remind readers that the 7-minute workout is not just about getting fitter but also about being able to move more in general.

Chapter 1: The Benefits of Doing the 7-Minute Workout

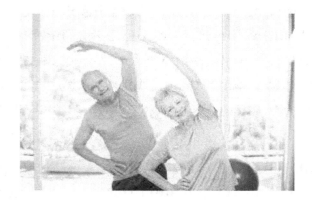

The 7-minute workout is beneficial in many ways.

The fact that the workout only takes seven minutes is great for working adults who do not have much time to work out but want to stay fit. This is also beneficial for children's after-school activities, as kids tend to be very busy and would not have the time nor patience to do a long workout. This is also beneficial because it requires only your body weight and no fancy equipment.

The 7-minute Workout could also be used to help individuals suffering from chronic diseases such as diabetes, hypertension, and heart disease by reducing their risk of developing certain diseases associated with sedentary lifestyles. It reduces the risk of developing other illnesses (e.g. obesity) that can lower your quality of life.

The 7-minute Workout is not just for adults; it is also beneficial to children and teens. It helps in fostering a healthy lifestyle early in life and ultimately lowering the risk of developing illnesses that are associated with sedentary lifestyles (e.g. heart disease, diabetes, obesity). Kids can do these exercises at home as often as possible because they only take seven minutes and they do not need expensive equipment.

The seven-minute workout is structured into four intervals. The workout has three different levels, each with their own workout routine.

I. Warm-up: Jumping jacks, High Knees, Butt Kicks and Star Jumps (each circuit for 30 seconds).

II. Strength Training: Squats (15 repetitions), Push-ups, Lunges (each circuit for 30 seconds). III. Core Strengthening: Crunches and Planks (each circuit for 30 seconds).

IV. Cool Down: Supermans and Back Extensions, Tricep Dips with a chair (each circuit for 30 seconds).

Benefits of doing the 7 minute workout to the old:

1) You will save yourself precious time in the mornings.

2) You will feel fresh and energized after your workout.

3) The workout is perfect for beginners.

4) It will help you build very lean muscle.

5) You can get very good results with this routine even if it is your first time working out.

6) It is a best way to maintain healthy weight.

7) It is an easy home workout, which requires just a pair of dumbbells, and a chin-up bar (or two chairs).

Gravity training utilizes the force of gravity as a resistance and does not require any special equipment or the purchase of expensive gym memberships.

Yoga is the practice of achieving physical, mental and spiritual balance through breathing, relaxation, and postures. Many people consider yoga as a way to reduce stress and improve overall health. Regular practice can be beneficial for flexibility, muscle strength, cardiovascular fitness, balance and coordination.

The 7-Minute Workout for Seniors has many benefits:

In order to improve performance in a physical activity it is necessary to do exercise. This does not mean that all exercise will increase performance in this activity it simply means it is necessary to do some exercise. Exercise can have many different benefits depending on the person's goals for their fitness program. In general exercise will strengthen our muscles and cardiovascular system which in turn will make us more fit. We often take for granted the many benefits we get from exercising. If you exercise regularly you will not only be healthier but happier as well. When we exercise our body releases endorphins which are said to make us feel good and happy. The endorphins also make us feel like having more energy too!

The 7-Minute Workout is said to be designed for seniors but can be beneficial to anyone who is a novice exerciser or has poor health, such as heart disease or diabetes. This workout consists of three rounds of seven exercises that should last about seven minutes in total. It is important to warm up before performing this workout and cool down after it as well. The author suggests that you should try to do this workout three times a week. The 7-Minute Workout for Seniors consists of 10 exercises. It takes only six minutes in total to do the circuit once. Perform one set of each exercise in the first minute and then one set of two exercises in the second minute, three sets of two exercises in the third minute and finally four complete rounds. These exercises are:

The core is a group of muscles that help stabilize your body during movement and keep it upright on both land and water. Strengthening your core muscles will help improve your performance in activities such as dancing, swimming, running or cycling. Core strengthening exercises usually target the lower back, upper back, abdominal muscles and hips.

The 7-Minute Workout for Seniors consists of three minutes of core exercises. The six exercises are:

The muscles in our body can be divided into two groups based on their location and function. Flexor muscles bend the joint and extensor muscles straighten it. There are some muscles that do both flexion and extension at the same time, such as the hip muscle. The 7-Minute Workout for Seniors consists of three minutes of strength exercises. These exercises target flexor and extensor muscles and help improve your performance in activities such as walking, running, swimming or golfing. The six exercises are:

The three strength training exercises are:

The last three minutes of this 7-minute workout is known as the cool-down and consists of three exercises. These exercises help relax your muscles after a hard workout :

These four sets together make up 6 minute circuit in a 7 minute workout.

The book gives many reasons why we should exercise and participate in different physical activities such as dancing. The author states that one of the best ways to achieve a healthy body is by reducing our risk of developing many illnesses such as heart disease, obesity, diabetes, osteoporosis and depression. The author states that it is also important to eat a healthy diet because the food we eat can help our muscles recover faster after exercising or help them grow. The author also claims that by improving our health we can save money on medical bills and also have better quality of life.

The 7-Minute Workout for Seniors has proven to be beneficial throughout many stages of life, but particularly when beginning a fitness program or being diagnosed with heart disease or diabetes as stated in the introduction. This workout has also been proven to maintain muscle strength as we get older which is very important because it can improve balance and reduce the risk of falling which is one of the leading causes of death for seniors. This workout is also beneficial before and after a surgery. It can help with rehabilitation after the surgery and it will also help you get back into shape faster. This workout can improve cardiovascular fitness, balance, coordination, bone density and muscle strength. The 7-Minute Workout for Seniors is also beneficial for individuals who have chronic diseases such as diabetes, osteoporosis or heart disease because it can help reduce your risk of developing other diseases associated with sedentary lifestyles such as obesity or cardiovascular disease.

The 7-Minute Workout is designed to be done at home, but you can do this workout almost anywhere: at the gym, in your dorm room or in a hotel room. There are no special equipment needed to do this workout except for the following (if you don't have them at home) It is recommended that anyone who has just started exercising should begin by doing the exercises in the circuit three times and then working their way up to five times. It is also suggested that you progress from one circuit to another by increasing your repetitions (e.g., three sets of 10 each exercise). In order to improve your cardiovascular fitness you can do exercises such as jogging, walking, or cycling. Since you will be performing three circuits of this workout it is suggested that you perform the cardiovascular exercise for 10 minutes. The author suggests that for each circuit you should work up to about 80 percent of your maximum heart rate and then decrease it in order to recover. It is also suggested that the cool down should last about 1-2 minutes. It is also important that you drink plenty of water throughout each day and eat a healthy diet in order for your muscles to recover faster.

Chapter 2: How to do the 7-minute Workout

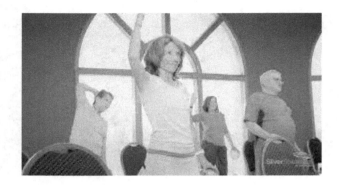

This introduces the reader to the different exercises that can be incorporated in the 7 Minute Workout. It describes a range of bodyweight exercises that can be carried out without any special equipment but with varying levels of intensity

For example:

1) Standard push-ups – performed on hands and toes on a hard surface such as a floor – can build strength, improve posture, and help prevent injuries. This is one of the most simple exercises that anyone can do anywhere at any time. This exercise can be made harder by performing a push-up on one's knees instead of the standard position.

2) Squats – performed in a standing position with the feet at hip distance apart and then bending down until the knee is at right angles or close to it. This will help to build strength in the core and lower body, as well as improving overall balance.

3) Lunges – performed in a standing position with one foot forward and one back. As you lunge, focus on keeping your upper body straight and upright with your weight on the heel of your front foot. This will improve overall strength in the legs, improve balance, as well as working out different muscles depending on which leg is used during the lunge.

4) Planks – performed with the body in a straight line and supported on the hands and toes. This exercise is designed to strengthen the core and increase overall flexibility.

5) Crunches – this exercise can be done by lying on your back with your knees bent and feet flat on the ground, or alternatively, for those who are more mobile, it can be preformed by sitting up with legs crossed to build strength in the core.

6) Raises – this is another simple abdominal exercise that anyone can do anywhere at any time. It involves simply drawing one's shoulders up towards their ears, holding for a few seconds and then lowering back down again.

This also focuses on the importance of exercise to the aging population, who are often perceived as a sedentary population who are not as active. However, close examination reveals that there is an active senior population in old age and it is important to recognise this and continue the activity into old age. Despite this, activity levels do start to fall off after around 65 years of age, so it is important for seniors to continue exercising despite many thinking that they don't need the exercise in their older age. This chapter also explains the difference between physical activity and exercise, with exercise referring to any intentional movement done with a specific goal.

The difference between physical activity and exercise are:

1) Physical activity is any activity done outside of work that requires energy to perform

2) Exercise is a physical activity that has a specific goal. E.g. running to lose weight, swimming to improve stroke technique

3) Physical activity can be unpaid e.g. gardening, walking with friends, walking to work

4) Exercise is paid for e.g. gym, swimming lessons, aerobics class

It gives a thorough overview of the benefits of physical activity for seniors and focuses on the importance of being active as part of a healthy lifestyle, through both exercise and daily activities. By giving examples it tries to raise awareness in people about the necessity of staying active as part of an overall healthy lifestyle and that growing old does not mean having to stop doing things one enjoys or is good for them in general.

If you're 60 or older, the thought of becoming frail, suffering injuries from falls, and losing your independence is often a real worry, even if it isn't already happening. Our body changes as we age—and often in ways we don't like. We naturally lose 1–2 percent of our lean muscle mass every year after the age of 50. This gradual loss of muscle and strength is barely noticeable at first—until we wake up one day surprised that our physical ability is not what it used to be.

What if I could show you how to reverse muscle loss and reclaim your strength, balance, and energy faster than you ever thought possible?

It doesn't matter if you're 60 or 100 years old, or if you've been active or inactive your entire life. It doesn't matter if you're currently walking miles every day or struggling just to get up from a chair. It doesn't even matter if your health is perfect or imperfect. This book will show you how to transform your body and your life, no matter who you are, irrespective of your current state of health and fitness.

The book explains the core principle of the program: 'Use it or lose it'. It explains why this is fundamental to both staying healthy and preventing falls as you age. It presents the science behind how exercise can decline with old age and how exercise can prevent or at least minimise these declines. Furthermore, it gives examples of what exercises one can do as part of their program to combat these declines in physical abilities.

It discusses why balance is important for an active life and also goes through a number of ways one can improve their balance. It also has an entire chapter dedicated to the importance of staying physically fit in order to prevent falls. This chapter goes through what causes falls, common myths about preventing falls and the science behind why exercises can help you stay balanced. It also gives examples of exercises that can be used as part of your program and how often you should do them in order to stay balanced. During the last few years there has been an increasing body of research on the topic whether brain training programs designed to improve cognitive functions such as memory, attention and decision-making are effective and reliable. The term does not include persons administered anesthesia or other psychoactive drugs while they are in an operating room, recovery room, intensive care unit or any other environment related to the practice of surgery or medicine. The term neurocognitive aging is the same as normal age-related cognitive decline. The main difference is that normal age-related cognitive decline is more global and diffuse, whereas neurocognitive aging involves areas of the brain that are more or less impacted than others.

Neurocognitive decline does not include gradual change in personality over time which happens with normal aging called "normal personality reorganization". Consequently, neurocognitive decline can occur independent of personality changes. One distinctive aspect of neurocognitive aging is that it substantially interferes with the individual's ability to pursue meaningful and purposeful activities during middle and late adulthood. As a result, the process of aging often leads to considerable disability and dependency in individuals who are otherwise physically healthy. Neurocognitive decline is not a disease. It is simply a natural process that everyone experiences as they age.

According to the research conducted by Eyal Shahar and colleagues on elderly individuals who regularly spent time outdoors, cognitive functioning was observed to be greater in those individuals compared to those who did not spend as much time outdoors. This was connected to activity of the hippocampus, which is an area of the brain associated with spatial knowledge, memory, and emotion. Other research has found that when elderly patients who suffered from Alzheimer's were exposed to nature for two months they showed visible improvements in brain functioning. This included increases in activity of the hippocampus, cerebellum, and superior parietal lobule, which are areas of the brain associated with memory. Staying physically active is important for everyone, but it's especially vital for older adults who are more at risk of falling and having other injuries. This book provides a series of 12 exercises that can be done in just 7 minutes and that will increase strength, improve balance, build coordination, and more. Each exercise takes only a few minutes to learn. Already in the first week of doing the program you will be able to see great results in your body, and over time you will transform your fitness level and your confidence level!

Chapter 3: Three Powerful Techniques to Make Exercise a Habit

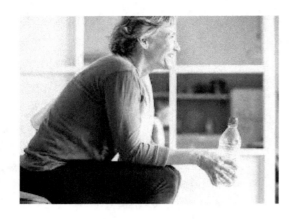

So you know from the previous 2 chapters that exercise is important and it will help you achieve your health, fitness and weight loss goals faster.

However, to make sure exercise becomes a habit, you need to use a specific approach. On this chapter I'll explain to you the 3 powerful techniques that will ensure your success. These techniques are: Decide what to exercise Focus on one thing at a time Implement the right rewards system

1. Decide What To Exercise This is so important! Don't just let yourself go or do what feels good at the moment. Instead, decide on the type of exercise program that you will do. For example, your goal is to lose weight, so instead of just running every day for 30 minutes, decide to do interval running. You may think interval training is just another way of exercising but it's not! If you want to gain more knowledge about interval training (and why I believe this type of

training is the best) read Born To Run by Christopher McDougall. So "decide what to exercise" doesn't necessarily mean you need to get a gym membership or equipment (although those things can help). Even if there's no gym nearby or you are too busy, all you really need are your body and your mind.

2. Focus On One Thing At A Time Decide what to exercise. You have to decide everything at once. So for example, if your goal is to lose weight and look better, decide that you will do the following: Interval running 3 times a week Weight training 3 times a week Yoga 1 time a week 15 minute meditation Daily water consumption of 2 liters Start with step 1! Don't worry about the others yet. It's important that you focus on only one thing at a time and when you've completed it, move on to the next one. So you may ask me: "How do I know which one to focus on first?" That's a great question. The answer is to ask yourself what's the most important for your situation. If you are overweight, it's very likely that exercise will help you burn more calories and thus lose more weight. So maybe put the interval running first and then move on to weight training later when you can fit it into your schedule. Decide what to exercise, this is half of the battle!

3. Implement The Right Rewards System The best thing about having a goal (like

losing weight) is not just reaching it but also achieving smaller rewards along the way. This will keep you motivated and push you to stick to your plan. You can also use these rewards to make yourself feel better about yourself! Here is a list of rewards that I recommend: Decide on the 1st reward you will give yourself (could be a new pair of workout shoes or a nice dinner) Make sure your rewards are limited (don't go overboard with them, choose something reasonable like two rewards for every 5 pounds) Find ways to enjoy these benefits, like eating a nice meal at the mall or window shopping

Now go out there and find a cool exercise program that's right for you. Make sure it's something you enjoy doing and can do regularly.

Technique 1: Habit Stacking

Habit stacking is a technique that will force you to do a series of habits. Our brain is lazy, which is good from one perspective, because once we've learned something it'll be easier for us to repeat it in the future. However, just like all other things, our brain needs some kind of stimulation so we stay on top of things. Habit stacking helps us with this by forcing us to initiate several habits at once and then take the actions needed to complete them.

One powerful application of habit stacking for exercise is a method called Run-Walk-Run .

What it is:

You alternate running with walking, so in other words you run and then walk. By doing this, you are able to exercise more efficiently and burn more calories.

How will this help me?

The answer to this question is really simple: if you walk more than you run, your heart rate and breathing will slow down instead of speeding up like when running. This means that your heart has to work less hard for the same amount of time. The result of this is that your body will burn fewer calories on a given period of time than if you were running all the time.

Technique 2: Conditioned Cues

This is an interesting technique that will allow you to prepare your mind for exercise and make it into a habit. It's very similar to how Pavlov's dog was conditioned to salivate in anticipation of food.

What is it?

You associate certain cues with exercising. For example, if you want to work out at the beach, then you may decide that when you start seeing the ocean, it's time for your run or walk workout. The idea is that once you start feeling that cue, your body (and your brain) will automatically prepare for exercise and you'll have a better chance of staying active throughout the day.

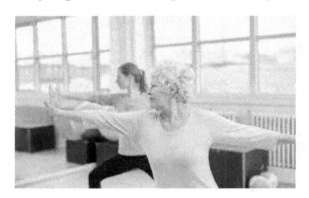

Technique 3: Intrinsic Reward Statements

This technique is somewhat similar to habit stacking but it's also a little bit different. The basic idea here is that you intersperse different activities into your workout. For example, instead of just running for 30 minutes, you can interleave jogging with jumping jacks. This will help you stay alert and active throughout the whole workout session.

Another example would be for weight training. Instead of just doing the same thing over and over again, you could do an exercise (like bench presses), then do something different (like bicep curls), then go back to bench presses and so on. This will keep your mind from getting bored and thus keep you more active throughout the workout session.

What is it:

This technique, pretty much like its name suggests, involves creating a visual representation of your exercise routine. This could be something like a poster with pictures to remind you of your workout plan for the week. Just seeing that reminder everyday can be enough to force you to act on it. Another option is to use an app or software program that helps you make the chart so you don't have to do the work yourself. There are two programs I really recommend: My Fitness Pal (fitnesspal.com) and Fitocracy (fitocracy.com).

How will it help me:

This technique is a bit different from the previous two. But personally I find it the most powerful of them all because you can use it no matter what your goal is. The idea behind this is that you create a goal and then you stick to it by posting it somewhere public where everybody can see. This way, if you don't start working towards your goal, people will notice and you'll feel bad about not taking action.Next time we'll be talking about how to make exercise a habit so stay tuned! In the meantime, keep on working out.

Key takeaways

Creating an exercise schedule that works best for you is not enough. That's why you need to learn how to make exercise a habit and start doing it without putting too much effort into it. I've outlined three techniques that will help you do just that:

1. Implementation Intentions

2. Habit Stacking

3. Visualization

There's one more technique you can use, which is a combination of the first two: First, make your schedule and then create an implementation intention to start implementing the schedule. This way you can make sure your schedule is not just sitting on a piece of paper but it's actually working for you.

Chapter 4: Great Results at Home with Little or No Equipment

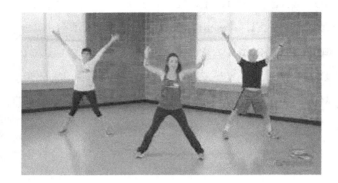

During the coronavirus pandemic, workout equipment flew off the shelves, with millions of people scrambling to put together a home gym because fitness centers were closing across the country. Equipment such as weights, exercise bikes, and rowers were out of stock for months. The good news is exercise can be just as effective without a gym or workout equipment. You can easily achieve the same results—or even better—exercising at home with little or no workout equipment using something called "functional training."

Functional Training

Functional training mimics activities or specific skills you perform at home, at work, or in sports to help you thrive in your daily life. This kind of training is effective because it uses different muscles simultaneously and also emphasizes core stability — the control of muscles around the abdomen and back that protect your spine when you move. For example, performing squats with a chair trains the same muscles you use when you rise from a chair, pick up an object from the ground, climb stairs, or hike up a mountain.

Many fitness and rehabilitation experts, including myself, have known for a while that functional training is the most effective way to train. Finally, the research is catching up with our observations. Functional training has now been shown in multiple studies to produce results that are superior to most other forms of exercise for diverse groups of people, including young military personnel, middle-aged females with low back pain, and (of course) older adults.14

One study demonstrated that high-intensity functional training was safe and effective for improving balance and independence in individuals aged 65 and older who had dementia and were living in nursing homes.15 Another showed that functional training significantly improved the golf swing and fitness level of golfers aged between 60 and 80 years old.16

By training your muscles to work functionally, you'll prepare your body to perform well in a variety of tasks that are important to your daily life—and you can do it at home with the aid of "equipment" readily available, such as a backpack filled with canned goods, to increase the difficulty level of exercise.

Exercising at Home

There are several additional benefits to exercising at home versus going to a gym:

• The ease and convenience of exercising at home removes demotivating barriers. You don't have to drive to the gym, change your clothes in a room full of strangers, or wait for workout equipment to free up.

• The gym can be an intimidating place for some older adults. But self-consciousness or fear of what others may think is not a concern with functional training at home.

• For older adults who don't function well enough to leave home without assistance, going to the gym can be difficult or impossible. Exercising at home is the only way for these people to improve strength, balance, and function.

• The price tag of a gym membership can be an obstacle for many older adults on fixed incomes. Cost is not an issue with workouts at home that require little or no equipment.

Combination Approach

The real secret to this program is the integration of higher-intensity training (discussed in the last chapter) and functional training, adapted for older adults. You won't find this combined approach to exercise for older adults in many other places, but it's a method that will allow you to safely and quickly achieve great results at home with little or no equipment.

You may be wondering at this stage why you couldn't just do something else that needs no equipment—such as walking—for exercise. It's certainly true that walking is another form of functional training that doesn't require equipment and can be good for your health, but in the next chapter I'll explain why walking alone isn't enough to reverse age-related muscle loss.

Key Takeaways

• You can easily achieve the same or even better results exercising at home with little or no workout equipment using "functional training."

• Multiple studies have shown functional training to produce results that are superior to most other forms of exercise for diverse groups of people, including older adults.

• The real secret to this program is the integration of higher-intensity training with functional training adapted for older adults. It will allow you to safely and quickly achieve great results at home with little or no equipment.

Action Steps

• Prepare yourself for exercising at home by making sure you have the following items handy:

o A backpack filled with heavy items (such as canned goods) for resistance.

o A pair of five-pound ankle weights.

• If you're a family member or a caregiver for an older adult you'd like to help with exercise, prepare them for exercising at home by making these items available.

• Only use a pair of five-pound ankle weights, and not heavier ones, when you exercise. Lighter weights are more comfortable and will allow you to perform the exercises with better form.

It is important to note that the risk of a heart attack or stroke is highest in the first three days following a sudden change in physical activity levels. Therefore, it is critical to speak with your doctor before starting an exercise program.

• It's best to begin with about 3 minutes of exercise per session and build up gradually over the next few weeks to as much as 10 minutes at a time.

• It's not necessary to do all twelve exercises every week—in fact, you may find that you feel more comfortable adding just two or three new exercises each week.

• Workout every day at home (ideally) or 3 days/week for optimal results from this program.

• It is important to incorporate a warm-up and a cool-down into your home workout to prevent injury and experience greater benefits.

• Perform each exercise with perfect form at least two or three times before moving on to the next exercise.

• Check with your doctor before starting this program.

• To maintain gains obtained from working out, it's vitally important to resist the urge to take breaks when you can easily fit in a workout routine.

What you need to know about training at home:

• It's common, especially in older adults, to experience some aches and pains after a workout. If this occurs, stick with the program, but cut back on the intensity of the exercise or change the duration of your workout until you can tolerate it well. For example, instead of doing 10 minutes of walking, do 5 minutes walking and 5 minutes of easy stretching.

• If you experience chest pain that is not relieved by medicine or does not go away within a few minutes after stopping exercise, it may be a sign of unstable angina (a warning sign for heart attack). Seek medical help right away.

• If you experience tightness, pain, or numbness in the area of your chest that does not subside within a few minutes, it may be a sign of a heart attack that is occurring right now. Seek medical help right away as this can cause sudden death.

• If you experience sudden dizziness or nausea while exercising and it does not go away within a few minutes after stopping exercise, it may be a sign of an inner ear disturbance—a warning sign for stroke. Seek medical help right away.

• If you have high blood pressure or a history of heart attack or stroke, consult with your doctor about starting this program slowly with lower-intensity exercise and shorter duration at first. I recommend that these individuals start by doing 3 minutes/day of exercise and progress gradually by adding 1 minute of exercise each week. When they can tolerate 10 minutes per day, they can return to the regular program.

• If you have osteoporosis, a history of broken bones, or if you have ever fainted due to low blood pressure, it is very important to talk to your doctor about having an exercise stress test before starting this program. Most individuals older than 60 who have had heart attacks or strokes should also have an exercise stress test.

• Seek a doctor's advice if you have had any of the following conditions and are considering starting this program: hypertension, heart condition (including an irregular heart beat), diabetes, chronic lung disease, joint problems, or smoking.

• If there is any doubt about your ability to exercise—due to health problems or medications you are taking—you should consult with your doctor before starting this program.

Chapter 5: The 7 Minute Workout for Seniors: Rest and Recovery

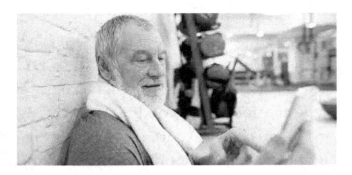

This chapter focuses on the rest and recovery aspect of the 7-Minute Workout. The author explains that using the seven minutes to work out is not enough and that a routine such as this must be complemented by adequate time spent in rest and recovery. The rest and recovery aspect of the 7-Minute Workout is made up of three phases: Early Recovery, Late Recovery and Active Recovery.

Early Recovery phase

In the Early Recovery phase, the author recommends that you should get off of the floor or out of the water and sit for a short period of time. Here you can even perform some gentle stretching if this is comfortable. If you exercise in a pool or at the beach, then you can simply stay in the water and float on your back for a few minutes. In this phase, it is recommended that you refrain from any intense exercises. It is said to be important to separate this from the Early Recovery phase and perform it about

twenty minutes after the workout is completed.

While moving into the Late Recovery phase, it is recommended that you perform energizing exercises such as arm circles or leg swings. This should be done for approximately 2-3 minutes after the workout has ended. It is also recommended that you continue your rest and try not to sit or lay down for long periods of time. The author suggests that you may want to begin performing gentle stretching at this point but stay away from Yoga or Pilates because they increase flexibility which can cause an imbalance in your muscles and joints. The Late Recovery phase should last about five minutes.

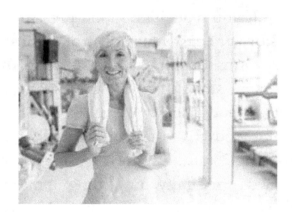

The Late Recovery phase

This is the most important phase of rest and recovery because this is when your body becomes ready for its next major stress or challenge. The author explains that we are not at a state where we need to be worrying about recovering our bodies in this case as we already have. It is said that during this time it can be important to get sufficient amounts of sleep because during sleep our body heals itself with increased blood flow. During sleep the blood flow to our brain increases by 50% and we achieve REM sleep in which our concentration levels are better and the brain consolidates memories.

Active Recovery,

This period of training is low intensity and consists mainly of aerobic activity such as walking or cycling to improve circulation around the body. The author explains that this should be done for 30–60 minutes. This helps return blood that has built up in our muscles after exercise back into the blood stream. If Active Recovery Phase is not followed, there is a danger of overtraining because after several days of hard training you will have fatigue which could lead to illness, injury or burnout.

When your muscles and joints are in the Early Recovery phase, you can try to strengthen your connective tissues with exercises such as yoga. By doing this the author says you can improve flexibility and prevent injury which could otherwise be caused by a weak or brittle muscle. The author states that performing yoga for a short 3 minutes after a Workout is enough to significantly increase circulation, heart rate and respiration which will enhance

recovery in addition to reducing stress and anxiety.

The second half of this chapter provides many different methods of how you can improve rest and recovery such as stretching, self massage, tapping and meditation. The final section of this chapter is titled "Yoga, Strengthening and Balance." The author explains how the practice of yoga (see Yoga) has proven to be beneficial for all ages. The author then explains how yoga can be incorporated into a 20 or 30-minute workout because we are all short on time and this is the main reason why the 7-Minute Workout for Seniors was invented in the first place.

The author explains that a good warm up should last 10–20 minutes and can include exercises such as walking, jogging, cycling, swimming or any other activity that gets your heart rate up. After this the author says that we should do a circuit of exercises for 7 minutes. The 7-Minute Workout for Seniors consists of 10 exercises that should be performed in a circuit style. In the first minute perform 1 set of each exercise and then in the second minute perform 2 sets, and so on until you reach 7 sets. The author states that it is possible to perform this workout in both a fasted state or after eating. The author then provides a table with each exercise listed along with the page number where it can be found and details about how much weight to use/how deep to go and also which muscles that exercise works out. The circuit consists of the following exercises:

The last exercise in this circuit is a plank. The author states that the plank is a good way to measure progress because it has no weight requirement and only takes ten seconds to complete. The author says that when you begin the 7-Minute Workout for Seniors this plank should be held for 15–20 seconds and you should work towards increasing it to 60–90 seconds. This second half of this chapter contains information about Yoga, Strengthening and Balance. The author explains how by practicing yoga you can strengthen your muscles, improve balance, relieve stress and have more energy at rest. The author also claims that practicing yoga will improve your flexibility. The chapter starts off with a description of Yoga. The author then explains how yoga can be incorporated into a 20 or 30-minute workout and how to do each movement correctly. The following yoga postures are described with pictures to help you see the correct form:

Next are all the exercises that you can use if you are not doing a yoga routine such as squats, lunges, push-ups, bridges, calf raises and planks. These exercises will help strengthen the muscles and increase bone density in your body. You can do this along with walking or any other aerobic activity because it is said that "muscle strengthening is key to improving muscular health. Strength training has been linked to delaying the onset of physical disabilities, which reduces the risk of falling and fracturing bones." The last section in this chapter is for Balance Exercises. The author then explains how "improving our balance can reduce our risk of falling, which is important as falls are one of the leading causes of injuries and death among older adults." By doing these exercises you will be able to get your muscles ready for challenging movements that you will perform if you take dance lessons or go hiking with friends.

Chapter 6: Tips for Family Members and Caregivers

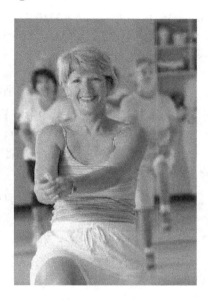

Older adults with memory issues or who lack the motivation to exercise will need help from another person.

Although we never want to force someone to exercise when they don't want to, persuasion is sometimes necessary because a persistent lack of movement leads to serious issues, such as debility, bed sores, and injuries from falls.

Older adults with memory issues or who lack motivation may have a difficult time starting and sticking with an exercise program. But I've found it becomes less challenging once exercise becomes routine, and changes in strength, balance, and energy become apparent after a few weeks.

The key to persuasion is a simple process I've created called the four Es: enthusiasm, empathy, encouragement, and ease. This process takes only a few minutes and has been effective with even my most exercise-resistant clients. Let's explore each step in detail.

Enthusiasm

Richard Simmons, the semi-retired American fitness instructor known for his eccentric and energetic personality, is a great example of enthusiasm at its best. It's difficult not to feel pumped up and motivated to move when you watch him.

So the first step in motivating someone is to be enthusiastic. Your enthusiasm is contagious, and it can shift another person's energy level and desire to exercise in powerful ways. To make enthusiasm work, you have to authentically feel it and express it in your words and body language.

Try to authentically feel and express enthusiasm in your voice, posture, gesture, and facial expression while saying something like, "Dad, it's time to exercise. It'll only take six minutes, and you'll feel great afterward. Let's do it!" If you encounter any resistance, move to the next step.

Empathy

The second step is to feel and express empathy: the ability to understand and share the feelings of another. It's important because a person is more likely to be open to your suggestions when they know you've understood and considered their perspective.

So to feel empathetic, you should know the common reasons why an older adult may not want to exercise: They may have lost hope that things will ever get better. They may be fearful that the aches and pains they experience daily will get worse if they exercise. They may feel constantly exhausted and don't know if they have the energy needed to exercise.

Whatever the reason, start by stepping into their shoes and feel what they may be feeling. Then express your understanding through your words and body language. Try to authentically feel and express empathy in your voice, posture, gesture, and facial expression while saying something like, "Dad, I can understand that you're feeling exhausted, and the aches that come with your age don't help. I also wonder if you've lost some hope that things can get better." It helps to pause for several seconds at this point to tune in to feelings that may be coming up for you and the other person. Then, move to the next step, which is to encourage the person.

Encourage

After feeling and expressing empathy, it's time to encourage the person to exercise.

For this to be effective, I suggest doing two things. First, understand the person's personal values and bring them into this step. A person's values can be things like determination or hope or respecting authority figures such as doctors. Second, remind the person of the benefits of exercise that are important to them. These benefits can be things like feeling more energized after exercising, gaining the ability to live more independently, feeling happier because they can avoid hospitalizations, or

having more energy playing with the grandchildren.

Whatever the reason for exercising, keep it positive, and express it with passion in your words and body language.

Use this step to authentically feel and express passion in your voice, posture, gesture, and facial expression while saying something like, "Dad, you always told us growing up that sometimes things will get worse before they get better, and having hope will get you through these times. It's no different getting your body working better through exercise. Remember how much you want to get back to gardening? What do you say?" If the person still isn't convinced to exercise at this point, it's time for the final step.

Ease

The fourth and final step is to ease into exercise. Use this when the previous steps haven't persuaded the person to take action. Your goal is to make exercise something the person can try for a few repetitions to see how it feels, knowing they can stop any time.

To make this step work, I recommend you first openly acknowledge that the person really doesn't want to exercise. Then suggest that they try just a few repetitions of one exercise to see how it feels. Tell them they can stop any time.

Perform this step with enthusiasm, and encourage the person to continue exercising after they've started. With enthusiastic encouragement, most people won't stop exercising once they've begun and may even surprise you with their new motivation.

Use this step to authentically feel and express enthusiasm in your voice, posture, gesture, and facial expression while saying something like, "I totally understand that the idea of exercise doesn't sit well with you right now, but let's just do five chair squats and see how it feels. I'll help you, and you can stop any time if you don't want to continue after that. Come on, let's start now."

As the person approaches the fifth repetition of the exercise, enthusiastically encourage them to continue by saying something like, "Wow, you're looking really strong! I'm amazed by how well you're doing! Keep going, I know you've got it in you!"

Applying the four Es takes only a few minutes and has been effective with even my most exercise-resistant clients. However, at times, nothing you do will persuade someone to exercise. It's best to yield to the person's wishes in these moments.

Fortunately, just two or three good workout sessions a week is enough to see improvements with this program in most adults. That may be all you will get out of someone who really doesn't like to exercise—but after a few weeks, they may be more motivated after noticing improvements in their strength, balance, and energy. So stay positive and be patient.

Key Takeaways

- The four Es can help persuade the person to exercise: enthusiasm, empathy, encouragement, and ease.

- The first step is to be enthusiastic. Your enthusiasm is contagious, and it can increase another person's desire to exercise. To make enthusiasm work, you have to authentically feel it and express it in your words and body language.

- The second step is to feel and express empathy: the ability to understand and share the feelings of another. A person is more likely to be open to your suggestions when they know you've understood and considered their perspective.

- The third step is to encourage. Understand the person's values and include them in your conversation, and remind them of the benefits of exercise that are important to them.

- The fourth and final step is to ease into exercise. Use this strategy when the previous steps haven't persuaded the person to exercise. The goal is to make exercise something the person can try for a few repetitions to see how it feels, knowing they can stop any time.

Action Steps

- If you're a family member or a caregiver for an older adult you'd like to help with exercise, practice the four Es a few times on your own to get comfortable with the method before using it to persuade them to exercise

Chapter 7: The Workout Routine

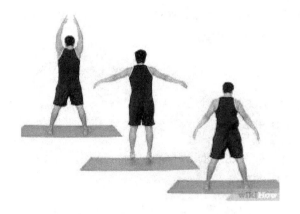

In this section, the exercise moves laid out in the previous chapter will be put together for a routine that will be suited to your fitness level. Determine your fitness level and take the fitness test in Chapter 4. Doctors recommend having at least 150 minutes of physical activity a week. Spread out over the week, that's 30 minutes of activity for five days. Workouts are great but you'll have to give your body time to adjust and recover. Two days of rest and recovery can be inserted midweek or during weekends. From 150 minutes, you'll build up to 225 minutes, and eventually 300 or more minutes a week. These routines aren't set in stone. As you progress and learn, and get used to the exertion, you'll have the confidence and the personal knowledge to mix and match exercise moves you feel would best suit your body's strength and endurance levels.

The plan is to do each level consistently for four weeks until you've increased your stamina and endurance, and could do more reps, more sets for longer periods. Before starting on any fitness routine, make sure that you've assessed your health and fitness functionality with the tests in Chapter 4. If you fall within the below average range, you'll start at the beginner level with a focus on 70% cardio to improve your stamina and 30% strength training. If you've an intermediate level result, the ratio is 60% cardio and 40% strength training. For those with results in the expert level, it'll be equal parts cardio and strength training. The routines outlined here are also adaptable to where you're most comfortable doing your exercises. A fifth of the exercises could be done outdoors - walking, cycling, and swimming. The rest can be done at home or at the gym. The exercise equipment needed is also minimal or easily adaptable with items readily found at home.

Work needs to be done to develop mobility and stamina if your fitness test shows below average results. Perform 15 minutes of stretching exercises to improve mobility and 15 minutes of simple cardio workouts.

Here's a sample stretching, strengthening, and cardio routine.

3 minutes of warm-up stretches

- Perform 2 times, Upper Back Stretch
- Perform 2 times, Chest Stretch

- Perform once on either side of the neck, Neck Stretch

- Perform 2 times, Sit and Reach Stretch

- Perform once for each leg, Inner Thigh Stretch

- Do 1 set of 16 reps, Shoulder Circles

- Do 1 set Hand Stretches

8 minutes of muscle strengthening & balance exercise

DAY 1

- 2 sets of 10 reps for each leg, Side Leg Raise

- 2 sets of 16 reps, Seated Shin Strengtheners

- 2 sets of 8 reps, Pliés

- 2 sets of 10 to 15 reps, Front Arm Raise

- 2 sets of 5 reps for each side, Side Bends

- 2 sets of 8 reps, Tummy Twists

- 2 sets of 10 reps for each leg, Knee Extensions

- 2 sets of 10 reps for each hand, Wrist Curls

- 4 sets of 15-20 steps, Toe the Line

- 2 sets of 10-second Flamingo Stands for each leg

- Perform 3 Clock Reaches for each side

DAY 2

- 2 sets of 10-second Flamingo Stands for each leg

- 2 sets of 10 reps, Side Leg Raise

- 2 sets of 10 to 15 reps, Front Arm Raises

- 2 sets of 5 reps for each side, Side Bends

- 2 sets of 8 reps, Tummy Twists

- 2 sets of 10 reps for each hand, Wrist Curls

- 2 sets of 10 to 12 reps, Bicep Curls

- 2 sets of 16 reps, Seated Shin Strengtheners

- 2 sets of 8 reps, Pliés

- 2 sets of 10 to 15 reps, Wall Push-Ups

- 2 sets of 10 reps for each leg, Knee Extensions

DAY 3

- 2 sets of 5 reps for each leg, Leg Lifts

- 2 sets of 15 reps, Seated Knee Lifts

- 2 sets of 10 reps, Knee Extensions

- 2 sets of 10 to 15 reps, Front Arm Raises

- 2 sets of 10 reps for each hand, Wrist Curls

- 2 sets of 10 to 12 reps, Bicep Curls

- 2 sets of 16-second Single Limb Stance with Arm for each leg

- Perform 3 Clock Reaches for each side

- 2 sets of 8 to 10 reps, Modified Burpees

- 2 sets of 5 reps for each side, Side Bends

- 2 sets of 15 reps, Seated Twists

DAY 4

- 2 sets of 5 reps for each leg, Leg Lifts

- Perform Bicycles for 30 seconds, rest, then go another 30 seconds

- 4 sets of 15-20 steps, Toe the Line

- Do 2 turns on the Speed & Agility Drill ladder

- 2 sets of 10 reps for each hand, Wrist Curls

- 1 set of 10 reps, Dumbbell Upright Row

- 2 sets of 10 to 15 reps, Wall Push-Ups

- Perform 3 Clock Reaches for each side

- 2 sets of 8 to 10 reps, Modified Burpees

- 2 sets of 8 reps, Pliés

- 2 sets of 16 reps, Seated Shin Strengtheners

DAY 5

- 2 sets of 10-second Flamingo Stands for each leg

- 2 sets of 16-second for each leg, Single Limb Stance with Arm

- 2 sets of 16 reps, Seated Shin Strengtheners

- 2 sets of 10 reps for each leg, Side Leg Raises

- 2 sets of 8 reps, Pliés

- 2 sets of 5 reps for each side, Side Bends

- 2 sets of 8 reps, Tummy Twists

- 2 sets of 15 reps, Seated Twists

- 1 set of 10 reps, Dumbbell Upright Row

- 2 sets of 10 to 15 reps, Wall Push-Ups

- 2 sets of 8 to 10 reps, Modified Burpees

15 minutes of cardio exercises
- 5 minutes marching in place

- 10 minutes of brisk walking

ALTERNATE CARDIO A

- a 15-minute bike ride or

ALTERNATE CARDIO B

- 5 minutes easy resistance on a stationary or elliptical bike

- 10 minutes medium resistance on a stationary or elliptical bike

2 minutes of cool down stretches
- Perform 2 times, Upper Back Stretch

- Perform 2 times, Chest Stretch

- Perform the cool down routine below:

1. March in place for 30 seconds.
2. Step your right foot forward to a lunge position and rest your hands on the middle part of your right thigh. Lunge forward taking caren't to let your knee go over your toes.
3. You should feel a bit of a stretch on your left calf. Hold the position for 16 counts. Switch positions and repeat step number 2 with your left leg.
4. Step your right foot behind and rest your hands on your hands on your right knee. Slowly bend from the waist pushing your buttocks backward and up.
5. You should feel a bit of a stretch on the back of your left thigh muscles. Hold the position for 16 counts. Switch positions and repeat step number 4 with your left leg.
6. March in place for 60 seconds. Stand with a wide stance and spread your arms upwards to stretch. Sweep your arms down to the side and raise them up again. Repeat this move for 8 counts.

Chapter 8: Is There an Ideal Diet?

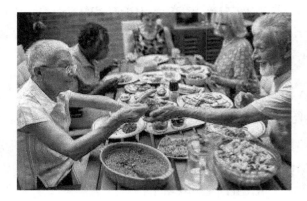

Walk into a bookstore and look for the section for books on diet. You will need time just to read the titles because the number of diets that are recommended is extensive. There are several reasons for this:

➤ Many people need help and guidance on weight loss and for managing conditions and illnesses: diabetes, heart disease, hypertension, cancers, immune disorders, and psychological problems among others.

➤ There is generally a belief that there is a magic diet, a silver bullet solution to lose weight, build muscle, cure disease, and live longer.

➤ · Diet is all about eating, and people generally take eating very seriously as evidenced by the size of the cookbook section at the bookstore.

Let's take a quick look at some of the diets that are popular today, but with the understanding that while there are responsible ways to help with weight control and prevent or alleviate certain

diseases, there is no single amazing diet that is the solution for everyone's problems. There is no "one size fits all" die because each of us has our own unique physiology, our own metabolic rate, our own sensitivities.

Popular Diets

Fasting has emerged recently as a way to health, happiness and a longer life, but you need to know that while the research involving worms and mice has been encouraging, the studies involving humans are mostly in the early stages. The more common approaches are intermittent fasting, conducted on a daily, repeating basis, such as the 16:8 fasting diet, which allows eating during an eight-hour period (e.g., 8 a.m. to 4 p.m.), and nothing to eat for the next 16 hours (4 p.m. to 8 a.m.). There are stricter versions, like 18:6. Alternatively, some try prolonged fasting, going for 24- or even 48- hour fasts, followed by a day of unlimited eating. People who practice this tend not to overeat on the non-fast days because their stomachs shrink a bit during the fast period,

➤ As a weightlifter seeking to build muscles, fasting diets are not advised for you.

Paleo diets harken back to paleolithic, simpler times when our distant ancestors were hunter-gatherers and ate "off the land," which means whatever they could find. This inspires diets today that avoid all refined and processed foods (which is commendable) and based on foods that our bodies evolved over millions of years to digest effectively.

A paleo diet limits foods like dairy products, grains and legumes, and potatoes that became available when farming and agriculture started around 10,000 years ago. Added salt is also avoided. Overall, the paleo diet is acknowledged as healthy and wholesome as long as the ratios of macronutrients are respected, and a diversity of foods is included so that adequate amounts of vitamins and minerals are included.

Keto diet, short for ketogenic, has a very specific objective: rapid weight loss through stimulation of fat burning. This is achieved by following a very high-fat, very low- carbohydrate diet, essentially replacing the carbs with fats. This results in a metabolic condition called ketosis, which is highly efficient in using stored and dietary fat, instead of carbs and stored glycogen, for energy. You burn fat; you lose weight. Another quality is the conversion of fat stored in the liver to ketones, which supply energy to the brain. Also, the keto diet has been shown to lower blood sugar and insulin levels, which may contribute to the prevention or reduction of diabetes and other disorders. Other benefits are a feeling of fullness (satiety) that reduces cravings to

eat or snack and improved mood. Studies of the longer-term effects of keto and other very low-carb diets are underway.

While the keto diet appears to be effective for weight loss, it may not include sufficient protein for building muscle mass; at least 30 percent of your diet should be protein.

Mediterranean diet. Let's conclude with a diet that is not only gaining broad acceptance, but it is the closest to the ideal diet everyone is searching for. It includes a wide range of wholesome and great-tasting foods, is affordable, is credited by the medical community as being heart-healthy, and may help slow the onset of many other diseases, from diabetes to cancer.

This diet is based on the practices of long-term residents of the Mediterranean Basin, including parts of Italy, Spain, and France, who tend to live healthier, longer lives. But importantly, these people practice a lifestyle that includes not only diet, but also being physically active all their lives, keeping their weight at normal levels, and having a positive attitude towards life.

The components of the Mediterranean diet:

➢ A variety of fresh vegetables, fresh and dried fruits, nuts, and seeds, whole grains and cereals, fish, lean meat in small servings (e.g., six ounces), moderate quantities of dairy (mostly as cheese), eggs, extra virgin olive oil, and wine, mostly red, consumed in moderation.

Whatever diet you choose, remember that as a weightlifter and builder of strength and muscle, you need sufficient protein in your diet, and you should select foods that are low in saturated fats. Avoid salty, processed foods, fried foods, and anything containing large amounts of sugar. The next section details the good and bad sources of foods.

Food Sources: Good and Bad

The types and sources of the three macronutrients have been discussed in detail, but to summarize, here is a quick checklist of the good and the bad. While this chapter has been devoted to helping you to understand the foods that are most beneficial to your health and to improve your level of physical fitness, build muscle and make you stronger, there are sources of carbohydrates, proteins, and fat that you should avoid. To help your dietary planning, we've listed both the recommended sources of your macronutrients and the foods that have been designated as undesirable and potentially harmful.

According to nutritionists at MD Anderson Cancer Center:

Recommended carbohydrates sources include:

➤ Dairy products, including milk, yogurt, and cottage cheese, but with a preference for low-fat or non-fat since full-fat dairy products are high in saturated fats and calories. Non-dairy substitutes made from soy, almonds, and oats are also good sources of carbs. Dairy products also provide high-quality complete protein.

➤ Vegetables, which can be eaten without limitation since they are low in calories and rich in vitamins and minerals. Select a variety of colors (green, yellow, red, purple) which will provide a diversity of micronutrients.

➤ Fruits are high in natural sugars (which is why they taste sweet) and micronutrients. Fruit should be eaten without added sugar and in natural, solid form to preserve pulp, which adds valuable fiber. Many juices have added sugar and the pulp has been removed.

➤ Beans, peas, and lentils, known as legumes, provide high levels of carbohydrates, plus fiber and many of the 20 amino acids that comprise protein.

➤ Whole grains, including whole wheat, rye, buckwheat, spelt, corn, and oats, are high in carbs and are excellent sources of vitamin B and fiber. Refined grains do not have these added qualities.

Carbohydrate sources to avoid:

➤ Refined flours and sugar, found in crackers, most breads, cookies, breakfast cereals, and sugar, in most fruit juices, soft drinks, most athletic performance beverages, and candy.

Recommended protein sources include:

➢ Beans, including black, pinto, and kidney beans, plus lentils and soy products. Except for soy, the proteins are incomplete and need supplementation with grains and cereals.

➢ Nuts and seeds, including nut butters (sugar-free versions).

➢ Whole grains, including quinoa, rye, wheat, spelt, corn, and soy, with the caveat that the amino acids do not comprise complete protein.

➢ Animal protein from meat, poultry, fish and seafood, dairy, and eggs.

Protein sources to avoid:

➢ Processed meats, like sausages, salami, bacon, frankfurters (hot dogs), and canned lunch meats.

➢ Consumption of lean red meats should be limited to 18 ounces per week.

Recommended fat sources include:

➢ Vegetable oils, especially extra virgin olive oil, avocado oil, and canola oil, and secondarily, oils from corn, sunflower, and safflower.

➢ Fatty fish, notably coldwater salmon, tuna, mackerel, and sardines.

➢ Flax seeds, chia seeds, avocados, and olives.

➢ Nuts and seeds, and again, natural nut butters, no sugar added.

Fat sources to avoid:

➢ Fried foods, which are made with refined flour and absorb large amounts of oils that contain trans fats.

➢ Animal sources, including full-fat dairy like milk, butter, yogurt, cream cheese, and the fats on meats and poultry.

➢ Vegetable oils from coconut and palm sources, shortening (used in baking), soft tub margarines, and most packaged baked goods (read the labels for fat content).

Now, on to Chapter 7 and dismissing some common misconceptions about working out, getting into shape, building muscles, and gaining strength when you are 60-plus.

Chapter 9: Motivation and Commitment

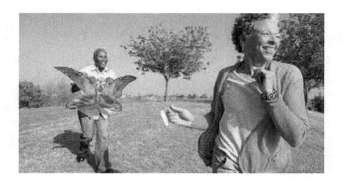

An important part of your long-term muscle and strength-building program is mental. Of course, it will be the weights, the reps, the sets, and the rests in between that will give you the lean muscle mass you want, but your state of mind will determine if you actually get started and if you will go the distance for the months and years of exercise it will take. Rome wasn't built in a day, and your impressive physique won't happen immediately.

The Motivation

In the initial chapter and at other points in this book, the importance of motivation was established as an incentive to getting your weightlifting and fitness program underway. No one can make you get into a regular, well-planned weightlifting program; you have to have the resolve and enthusiasm to take charge of your body, your health, and your appearance:

➤ If you have read this far, chances are good that you get it, "you're in."

➤ You imagine yourself lifting the barbells and dumbbells, doing the push-ups and pull-ups, the planks, the squats, and the splits.

➤ You feel committed to cardiovascular conditioning to help melt the extra pounds while you invest in your health and longevity.

➤ You feel better looking in the mirror in anticipation of the bigger, defined muscles you are going to build.

The Commitment

But will you have the determination and discipline to go the distance, to continue regularly with your bodybuilding and strengthening practices? Motivation is important at the beginning, but you need to have the discipline to stick to the routine even on days when you just don't have the drive, when you say, "I'll do it tomorrow."

You need to transcend the forces that hold you back, to break free of the constraints, and be committed no matter how tired or uninspired you are at that moment. Only then can you keep on track to meet your fitness and strengthening goals.

Commitment to succeed as a weightlifter, who builds muscle, who loses fat and excess weight, starts in the mind, which is the most effective and persuasive tool that will help you achieve your bodybuilding objectives. A positive attitude and the determination to work through the toughest movements will carry you through the worst of it with grit. Those who fail to make it, who give up, who quit, may be tough physically but don't have the mental toughness. Remember that your body will follow your mind.

Successful weightlifters at every level of training have developed positive thoughts to get themselves to the gym, to pick up the first weight of the session, to get through it with a full effort, no matter how tired or busy they were. You can adopt these thoughts, make them yours, let them carry you to the workout, and through the work, every time.

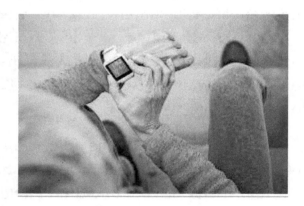

Positive Reinforcements

1. I'll just do a half-workout today, take it easy.

This works when you're tired and helps to get you started. In almost every case, once you get started and warmed up, you get into the movements, do all the reps, and go all the way. It's a little psychological game that you can play on

yourself, and somehow it continues to work time after time. As it has been said, "just showing up is 90 percent of success," so just get those workout shoes and shorts on, get to a machine or a weight, and start out slowly. You'll warm up and keep going.

2. The solo mountain climber's focus and discipline.

When you are heading up the side of Yosemite's El Capitan, climbing without ropes or tools, there is no looking up or down, no thinking about what's coming or how hard it will be. The same applies to weightlifting when the only thing that matters is what you need to do at that moment: focus on the now. Another advantage of being in the moment while working out is the clearing of your mind, in a meditative way, so that all distractions are ignored. You will be calmer, and by paying close attention, your form and posture will be better, and you will be less likely to cause an injury.

3. The mirror, the scale, and the tape measure.

The numbers don't lie, exaggerate, or try to please your ego. They are the reality that will testify to the depth and duration of your commitment to building your body, getting your weight where it belongs, and getting that gut flatter. Start with a benchmark set of measurements, and check in every week.

Look at yourself in the mirror without criticism or disappointment and just take notice of how your pecs (chest muscles) and abdominals look: a little soft, a layer of fat. Same for the arms and legs. Weigh yourself before breakfast, and write down the number each week, or daily if you prefer. Same for the tape measurement. Over time, you will see and record progress, and that will help solidify your commitment to your long-term objectives.

Inspirational Quotes

1. "Tough times don't last, but tough people do." — Richard Shuller (2020).

This quote applies to all aspects of life but has found special appreciation among professional lifters who push to their absolute limits. But especially for you as you are beginning weightlifting and conditioning, there are times when it isn't fun, like that last pull-up or barbell curl. Your thighs may be burning after three sets of squats or splits, and that last set of dumbbell rows may have you breathing pretty hard. But every time the set is over, and the rest begins, the pain and burning feeling subsides, and the workout always ends with a feeling of work well done, a sense of satisfaction. You are tough and getting tougher.

2. "To be a champion, you must act like a champion." — Lou Ferrigno (2020).

Lou Ferrigno, a champion weightlifter who played the Incredible Hulk, contributed to this recommended mindset because he believes that strength comes from within. A championship attitude is attainable by all of us if we believe in ourselves and envision the well-muscled, well-defined body we are working to achieve. But it goes further: If you want to become a well-built bodybuilder, you need to work out like one. Positive thinking is essential to motivate and inspire you, but without hard work and the determination to give it your all, positive thinking is just a dream.

3. "Don't wish it were easier. Wish you were better." — Jim Rohn (2020).

The thought leads us to expect that the workout, the lifting and pulling, the squatting and dipping, needs to be intensive, to challenge us. That leads to the realization that if it's easy, it's not being done right. You need to work to challenge your muscles to the point that muscle cells and fibers are damaged and need to self-repair through hypertrophy. The attitude that will carry you from passive to proactive is the recognition that it's a simple formula: strength is directly proportional to the effort that is invested in each workout. Of course, a hard workout can be followed in two days by a less intensive workout to aid recovery, but then be sure to make the next workout more intensive. It will pay off in the long-term.

4. "It never gets easier. You just get stronger." — Unknown (2020).

The idea is to add weights progressively when you can handle more without reducing reps, sets, or rest intervals. For example, head over to the dumbbell rack, and pick up a heavy weight you can do just one rep of a bicep curl or at most two. Do you wish you could do more reps? Find the weight you can lift or curl for eight reps and have the patience and confidence to know that in a reasonable time, with discipline, you will advance gradually from the lighter weight to the heavier ones and beyond. Just follow the basic practice of lifting weights that max out at eight to 10 reps, do the three sets, and be sure to rest between sets and between workouts.

5. "You have to be at your strongest when you're feeling at your weakest." — Unknown (2020).

This inspiration encourages weightlifters and cardio athletes to reach deep inside for the strength that they know is there. Imagine that you are a runner who is training for a marathon or other long-distance competition. The only time you can train is early in the morning before work, even in the cold and dark of winter. You need to roll out of bed at 5:30 a.m., wash your face, put on your running shoes, head outside, hit the road, and run into a biting cold headwind. What does it feel like to go through this, day after day, for months? This is what inner strength is all about, and it illustrates, in the extreme, what someone chooses to do to reach an objective. You probably will not have to work out under such an extreme condition. You'll be indoors, warm, lifting weights you can manage, and working to a reasonable, yet difficult peak of effort. But think of that runner in the dark, cold, early morning, and let it carry you to a better effort each day.

Chapter 10: Questions and Answers

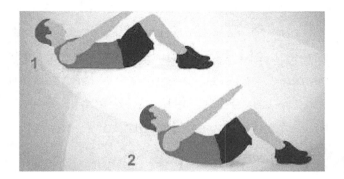

In order to stay fit the authors of the 7-Minute Workout suggest that you do this workout three times a week. The best time for you to do this workout is probably before or after breakfast, lunch or dinner. Even though you will only be performing circuits 2 and 3, it is suggested by the author that you consider doing circuit 1 too in order to warm up gradually.

The 7-Minute Workout for Seniors is a very beneficial workout routine for anyone. It is especially beneficial for people who are just beginning to exercise or individuals who have been diagnosed with heart disease, diabetes or osteoporosis. It is beneficial for people who are just beginning to exercise because it will help them become more fit and healthy. It is beneficial for people who have been diagnosed with heart disease, diabetes or osteoporosis because it can help reduce their risk of developing other diseases associated with sedentary lifestyles such as obesity or cardiovascular disease. This workout can also be used to improve muscle strength, balance and coordination. The 7-Minute Workout for Seniors is a great workout routine for individuals who are just beginning a fitness program or persons who want a simple and easy workout routine that helps them stay fit.

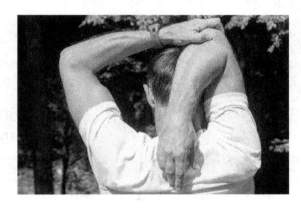

How to Improve Your Performance:

1) Always remember that you should warm up before doing any exercises.

2) The 7-Minute Workout for Seniors consists of four sets of exercises. For each set do 3 minutes (or 5 minutes in case you are doing circuit 2) with no rest in between the exercises.

3) The warm up should last about five minutes. It is recommended that you pick exercises that make your muscles feel a slight burning sensation and that also help you warm up slowly.

4) The 6 exercises consist of 1 minute, 2 minutes, 3 minutes and 4 minutes respectively. In order to learn more about how to do these exercises it is suggested by the author to check out the book titled "The 7-Minute Workout."

5) The cool down consists of three exercises and should last about two minutes.

6) You should drink plenty of water every day. At least one liter will be sufficient for the average person.

7) Eat a healthy diet to ensure adequate supplies of protein, carbohydrates and fats for your muscles. Also, eat plenty of different fruits and vegetables to ensure that you will get all the vitamins and minerals you need.

8) Plan to work out at different times in your week so you won't become bored or irritated by this workout routine. The book also suggests that you find a friend with similar goals as you do to help motivate yourself to include a fitness routine in your life regularly.

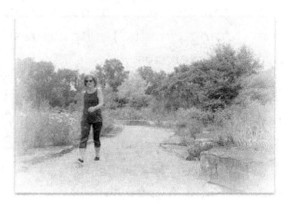

Questions and answers on the 7-minute workout for the seniors:

1. Can men do this workout?

This workout is be particularly beneficial for men. By doing this workout regularly the author of the book claims that it can help prevent heart disease and diabetes as well. This routine has also been proven to maintain muscle strength as we get older which is very important because it can improve balance and reduce the risk of falling which is one of the leading causes of death for seniors.

2. What are some other benefits of doing this workout?

This particular routine is good because it helps you improve your balance, coordination and bone density. It also helps you strengthen your cardiovascular fitness, muscles balance, coordination, bone density and muscle strength.

3. How many sets of exercises do I need to do?

The book suggests that you should do three sets of each exercise for about a minute. You also should perform each circuit three times before progressing to the next one. Progressing from one circuit to another by increasing your repetitions (e.g., three sets of 10 each exercise). The warm up should last about five minutes and you should work up to about 80 percent of your maximum heart rate and then decrease it in order to recover. It is also suggested that the cool down should last about 1-2 minutes. It is also important that you drink plenty of water throughout each day and eat a healthy diet in order for your muscles to recover faster.

4. Does the 7-Minute Workout for Seniors put a lot of pressure on my joints?

This workout routine is designed to be gentle for your joints because it is low impact and no knee or ankle weights are required.

5. How much space do I need to do this workout?

Since the 7-Minute Workout for Seniors consists of only three exercises that can be done at home or in other small places, it will not take up much space at all! It is very easy to do this workout routine.

6. What is the difference between circuit 1 and 2?

Circuit 1 consists of exercises that target your muscles and help them recover after performing other exercises. Circuit 2 consists of strength training exercises that target flexor and extensor muscles in order to improve your performance in activities such as walking, running, swimming or golfing.

7. Will I get bored doing this workout routine?

It is recommended by the author to use different times in your week for working out so you won't become bored. You may also want to find a friend with similar goals as you do to help motivate yourself.

The 7-Minute Workout for Seniors is a very beneficial workout routine for anyone. It is especially beneficial for people who are just beginning to exercise or individuals who have been diagnosed with heart disease, diabetes or osteoporosis. It is beneficial for people who are just beginning to exercise because it will help them become more fit and healthy. It is beneficial for people who have been diagnosed with heart disease, diabetes or osteoporosis because it can help reduce their risk of developing other diseases associated with sedentary lifestyles such as obesity or cardiovascular disease. This workout can also be used to improve muscle strength, balance and coordination. The 7-Minute Workout for Seniors is a great workout routine for individuals who are just beginning a fitness program or persons who want a simple and easy workout routine that helps them stay fit.

– This book will benefit you because it will help you improve your health by reducing your risk of developing many illnesses. The seven exercises contained in this book will help relax the muscles after a hard workout and also improve your cardiovascular fitness, balance, coordination, bone density and muscle strength.

- This workout is very beneficial because it does not take up much space at all! This routine consists of three sets of 6 exercises in order to be completed within seven minutes. It is very easy to do this workout routine. It can be done at home, the gym or even in a hotel room.

- This workout routine will help you improve your cardiovascular fitness because it contains exercises that target your muscles and help them recover after performing other exercises. Also, this routine helps relax the muscles after a hard workout and also improves your cardiovascular fitness, balance, coordination, bone density and muscle strength.

- This workout routine will help you stay fit because it can help prevent heart disease and diabetes. It can also develop your muscles strength as well.

- This routine helps improve muscle strength, balance and coordination. This workout also has been proven to maintain muscle strength as we get older which is very important because it can improve balance and reduce the risk of falling which is one of the leading causes of death for seniors.

- The 7-Minute Workout for Seniors consists of four sets of exercises that are all targeted for different parts of the body such as the chest, back, shoulders, arms, hips and thighs or legs. The warm up consists of three exercises in order to be completed within five minutes. The 6 exercises of this routine consist of 3 minutes, 4 minutes, 1 minute and 2 minutes respectively. In order to learn more about how to do these exercises it is suggested by the author to check out the book titled "The 7-Minute Workout."

- The cool down consists of three exercises and should last about two minutes.

- This workout routine has also been proven to maintain muscle strength as we get older which is very important because it can improve balance and reduce the risk of falling which is one of the leading causes of death for seniors.

- Information about why you should drink plenty of water everyday in order for your muscles to recover faster.

- Eat a healthy diet that provides you with adequate supplies of protein, carbohydrates and fats. Also eat plenty of different fruits and vegetables to ensure that you will get all the vitamins and minerals you need.

- Mix up your workout routine. Make sure that you plan to work out at different times in your week so you'll never get bored or irritated by this workout routine.

– You should drink plenty of water every day and eat a healthy diet in order for your muscles to recover faster.

Conclusion

This workout routine will improve your health by reducing your risk of developing many illnesses such as cardiovascular disease, osteoporosis and diabetes. This workout will help relax the muscles after a hard workout and also improve your cardiovascular fitness, balance, coordination, bone density and muscle strength. This program is very beneficial because it does not take up much space at all! It can be done at home, the gym or even in a hotel room.

This workout routine will help you improve your cardiovascular fitness because it contains exercises that target your muscles and help them recover after performing other exercises. Also, this routine helps relax the muscles after a hard workout and also improves your cardiovascular fitness, balance, coordination, bone density and muscle strength.

This workout routine will help you stay fit because it can help prevent heart disease and diabetes. It can also develop your muscles strength as well. This routine helps improve muscle strength, balance and coordination. This workout also has been proven to maintain muscle strength as we get older which is very important because it can improve balance and reduce the risk of falling which is one of the leading causes of death for seniors. The 7-Minute Workout

for Seniors consists of four sets of exercises that are all targeted for different parts of the body such as the chest, back, shoulders, arms, hips and thighs or legs. The warm up consists of three exercises in order to be completed within five minutes. The 6 exercises of this routine consist of 3 minutes, 4 minutes, 1 minute and 2 minutes respectively. In order to learn more about how to do these exercises it is suggested by the author to check out the book titled "The 7-Minute Workout."

This cool down consists of three exercises and should last about two minutes.

This workout routine has also been proven to maintain muscle strength as we get older which is very important because it can improve balance and reduce the risk of falling which is one of the leading causes of death for seniors.

This workout routine has also been proven to maintain muscle strength as we get older which is very important because it can improve balance and reduce the risk of falling which is one of the leading causes of death for seniors.

This workout can help prevent heart disease and diabetes as well. It can also develop your muscles strength as well.

This workout routine will help strengthen your cardiovascular fitness, balance, coordination, bone density and muscle strength. Also, this routine helps relax the muscles after a hard workout and also improves your cardiovascular fitness, balance, coordination, bone density and muscle strength. This workout routine will help you stay fit because it can help prevent heart disease and diabetes. It can also develop your muscles strength as well.

The 7-Minute Workout for Seniors is a very beneficial workout routine for anyone. It is especially beneficial for people who are just beginning to exercise or individuals who have been diagnosed with heart disease, diabetes or osteoporosis. This exercise program is very beneficial because it does not take up much space at all! The exercises that are contained in this book will help improve your health by reducing your risk of developing many illnesses such as cardiovascular disease, osteoporosis and diabetes.

The 15-Day Men's Health Book of 15-Minute Workouts

By

Lil Ron

Table of Contents

Introduction

The 15-minute workout is a revolutionary idea. Most of us have been taught that a good workout takes 45 to 60 minutes, three or four times a week. But the benefits we get from the time spent exercising last only as long as we can push ourselves—and sometimes even less than that. Even those who exercise six days a week for 50 minutes each time rarely lose weight, build muscle or gain strength to any significant degree because their bodies adapt quickly to the demands they are placing on them. That's why I've developed this 15-minute program so you can get stronger, leaner and healthier without having to spend hours at the gym. You'll get leaner, stronger and better at burning off body fat—and you'll do it in less time than it takes to watch an hour-long TV series.

The 15-minute workout is based on simple exercise science. Researchers have known for decades that our bodies adapt quickly to the demands we place on them through exercise. When that happens, we stop getting as much benefit from the workouts we're doing. It's a concept called overtraining or spiking cortisol levels: The stress of regular workouts increases your cortisol levels, which makes you tired when you should be energized. Over time, you will stop seeing progress because your muscles will begin to stop responding to the training. The only way to overcome this adaptation is to keep increasing the intensity of your workouts—and that can spell trouble for your body.

Even high-intensity interval training— the kind of workout where people alternate periods of strenuous exercise with periods of rest—will only give you a couple of weeks of results before your body adapts. You'll get stronger, but you'll also get leaner and faster, and then…nothing.

Why? Because one way our bodies store energy is by enhancing its sensitivity to insulin, which helps it use fat as fuel. This adaptation is good for endurance activities like running or biking, since it helps your body get energy from stored fat. But it's not so good if you want to lose weight and burn body fat. The only way to overcome this adaptation is to keep increasing the intensity of your workouts—and that can spell trouble for your body.

The 15-minute workout works differently from traditional training because it takes advantage of what exercise scientists call the "pump effect" and "metabolic chaos": short bursts of intense activity followed by brief spurts of rest—all performed in 15 minutes or less. During and immediately after a workout, your body is flooded with stress hormones that boost your metabolism and increase fat burning. The 15-minute workout also keeps cortisol levels from spiking, which means you'll feel energized for hours after you exercise.

The 15-minute workout will give you a leaner, stronger body and a calmer mind—but it's important to realize that it won't give the same benefits as those long workouts you're used to. You won't see the same results in terms of strength and endurance because your body won't have enough time to adapt to the increased intensity. The good news is that most of this adaptation occurs in the first 15 minutes of your workout, and after that, you can just focus on having fun, getting healthier and feeling better.

The magic combination for the 15-minute workout is a mix of intense weight training and fast intervals of cardio. I have designed two different programs based on these principles—one for total-body leanness (which includes a full-body circuit) and one for building strength. Both use simple exercises you can do with a barbell for weight training, a pair of dumbbells at home or nothing more than your own body weight.

Chapter 1: The Science of 15-Minute Workouts

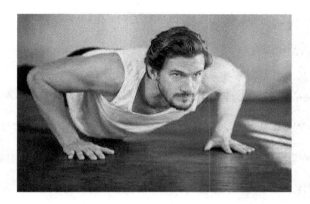

The best exercise, the most effective way to lose weight and get lean and healthy, takes place in the first 15 minutes of your workout. By "best" I mean that this type of workout is more effective than longer workouts because it boosts your body's metabolism and helps you burn fat. And by "least effective," I mean that workouts over an hour turn out to be counterproductive for most people, especially those who want to lose weight and build muscle. To be clear, this doesn't mean any exercise is better than no exercise. It just means that the kind of workout that offers the best results in the shortest period of time takes place in the first 15 minutes of your training sessions.

Advantages Over Traditional Workouts

1. It increases your metabolism and burns fat for hours after you exercise.

2. It keeps cortisol levels from spiking, which means you'll feel energized for hours after you exercise.

3. It's more effective in terms of building cardiovascular fitness than longer, less intense workouts (though if you get out of breath or lightheaded during your workouts, take a break and have a glass of water).

4. It leads to better weight loss than longer, less intense workouts because it helps you burn more fat in the hours following your workout (this point is debatable; see Chapter 7).

5. Your muscles respond positively to this type of workout with visible results; your body begins to shape up within two weeks.

6. It is more effective than longer, less intense workouts in terms of increasing muscle strength and endurance.

7. It keeps you focused on the workout itself, so you don't waste time worrying

about what you're wearing or how much time the guy next to you lifts weights.

8. It's perfect for busy people who can't commit to longer exercise sessions (but even those who can devote an hour or more to their workout will benefit from including shorter sessions in their week).

9. It improves your mood and mental health because it boosts endorphins and helps reduce stress levels—even during a stressful day at the office.

Disadvantages Over Traditional Workouts

1. It is tough for beginners.

2. It takes up more time in your day than longer, less intense workouts do (though you can incorporate it into your busy life without much fuss).

3. It's not easy to stay motivated; you can feel like you're not doing enough in the beginning when your body is still adjusting to this type of training.

4. Some experts say shorter workouts aren't an effective way to build muscle, but the research I've cited tells a different story.

5. It can be very hard on your joints and spine.

6. It places a lot of stress on your body, which may lead to injury.

7. You're going to feel sore the next day (which is why this type of workout works best if you plan it for before work or on weekends).

8. You risk overtraining—doing too much too soon—which could leave you vulnerable to injury and burnout.

9. It might actually make weight loss harder because some studies show that working out intensely boosts your appetite.

10. Some people get bored doing shorter workouts, but you can switch up your routine to help stop this from happening.

11. You're more susceptible to skipping a workout or falling off the fitness wagon.

12. You may lack the energy to perform other activities in your day-to-day life, which is not what you want if you're trying to be healthy!

13. Some short workouts don't offer all of the health benefits that they claim (or any at all).

The most effective way to make sure you're benefiting from your workout regimen is to do workouts that are 30 minutes or longer. This is why an hour-long session at a gym, yoga studio, or fitness class works best - it takes about fifty minutes for your brain and body to be engaged enough to use the movements effectively while you're building endurance and strength. If you notice yourself struggling the first time you try something new, stick with it and don't give up until you can reap all of the benefits of the workout. And if you find yourself struggling with motivation, try pairing up with a friend! You can motivate each other; plus, research shows we work out more frequently when we have a buddy.

The length of your workout matters because it determines what is happening in your brain and body. Shorter workouts, even if they are intense, won't give you the same benefits as longer workouts. Even if you feel like you're getting leaner and stronger with your short workout, it could be that the change is not due to the workout improving your muscle tone or endurance - it might just be that your body is getting better at burning off fat and conserving energy.

You might think that some forms of exercise are more effective than others, but the duration of a workout is not what you should be focusing on. What really matters is that you participate in a workout that gets your heart rate up, improves your endurance and works your muscles. The type of training most people use to "get in shape" at gyms these days falls into two camps: interval training and resistance training. The problem with these two types of training is that they can be very hard on your body if performed too frequently over too long a duration. The interval training that fitness junkies are so fond of doesn't work for everyone—especially if you're new to the activity or have a bad hip. Resistance training is all about strength-building, which is why I designed the resistance program at FitnessBlueprint.com. It's one thing to get stronger, but why focus on it when endurance and fat-burning are your real goals? That's why I created a workout that focuses on fat burning and building muscular endurance without putting your body through hard intervals of cardio or stressful resistance training. To do it, you'll have to keep your heart rate up and your muscles working, but you don't have to put your body through tough intervals over and over again. The rest of this book will explain the science behind this exercise program—and how it can help you get leaner, stronger and fitter in just 15 minutes a day.

Chapter 2: Maximizing Your Weight-Training Workouts

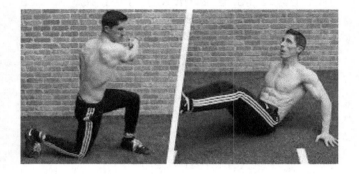

The best weight-training sessions last about 45 to 60 minutes, and they're designed to help you build lean muscle mass. Of course, that's not what we're going for. Our goal is to lose fat and improve our health, which is why I have designed a set of 15-minute workouts that will increase your metabolism and burn fat after each workout. These workouts are less intense than those traditional weight-training sessions that last an hour or more, and they don't require the same amount of time from you. You don't need to go to the gym and spend hours on exercise machines. You can lift weights using your own body weight, or you can use barbells and dumbbells you have at home. The workouts are simple, but that doesn't mean they're easy. To make them

effective, you'll need to push yourself—and work through that discomfort you might feel if this is your first time doing a workout like this or if it has been a long time since you have done a good weight-training session. I designed this program to help build muscle mass using basic barbell exercises that work every muscle in your body - including your chest, back, shoulders, abs and legs. Your muscles will be responding to this type of training within two weeks, and you can expect that they will change in terms of appearance and performance. Not everyone wants to look like a bodybuilder, but most people want to look better. And this program—which takes place over just seven days—will help you do just that. You'll gain more muscle and lose more fat than you would with an hour-long, traditional workout. And even though this program is focused on building muscle, it will help you burn calories through the work your muscles do. It doesn't matter if you want to lose five pounds or 50—every workout you do shapes your body in some way. This program is for everyone because it uses compound exercises that work multiple muscles at once. If you are very out of shape, the 15-minute workouts will help you burn calories, improve your endurance and lift more than you ever have before. If you are already in good shape but want to get even stronger or more toned, this program will help. If your goal is to just build muscle and stay healthy, this is the program for you. Every workout will help you get stronger, which is what building muscle mass is all about. And you can expect to start noticing visible results within the first two weeks. Your muscles will be much firmer, your biceps will be more defined, your abs will be more pronounced and your legs will look leaner. If you already have some muscle mass or you spend the time to really work out those areas that need it, you can expect to see a difference in how your body looks in about six weeks. There is no such thing as spot reduction - where one area of your body (your butt, for example) gets smaller while another part (like your thighs) gets bigger - but this program does help promote lean muscle mass throughout the entire body. Every workout session burns calories and elevates the metabolism for hours after you've finished exercising. You'll also notice that your clothes fit better because you're leaner, and there will be fat burning 24/7.

This workout will help you create a calorie deficit - the difference between the calories you eat and the calories you burn off. The more time passes, the bigger that calorie deficit gets, which means you lose more weight faster. If your goal is to lose about 1 to 2 pounds per week, this workout will help you get there. Whether this is your first weight-training program or not, each session should feel just as intense as it does for someone who is just starting out at the gym. If you aren't feeling the burn or you are feeling fatigued, you are not pushing yourself hard enough. Push through your workouts. Every time you work out, you should be able to do more of the exercises than the last time.

Repeat each set of exercises twice. You can do each set back-to-back or rest 1 to 3 minutes in between before moving on to your next set. Rest 1 to 3 minutes between each round, and complete four rounds in total. Rest 1 day before moving on to the next workout session.

1. Chest Press

This exercise targets your pectoralis major, and it's a great way to build your chest if you are new to weight training or have been away from the gym for awhile. To do it, place a barbell on your upper back. You can use an Olympic bar or an EZ curl bar. Step underneath the bar and squat down low while holding onto its ends. Stand up straight while holding the bar with both hands at shoulder width.

2. Rear Deltoid Flyes

This is another great exercise for beginners because it doesn't require much knowledge about form or equipment. All you need is a bench and some dumbbells. Sit on the edge of the bench with your back facing the ceiling. Grab one dumbbell and rest it on your chest. Lower it out to the side while keeping your arms straight and elbows

close to your body. Slowly bring it back up, squeeze your chest muscles and repeat for 10 reps on each side.

3. Triceps Dips

This exercise targets the triceps, which are some of the largest muscles in your upper arms. To do them, place a chair or bench so that it is standing behind you high enough that you can comfortably bend over and rest your weight on it without falling off. Place your hands on the edge of the bench with your fingers pointing towards you. Bend your legs under you and lower yourself until you feel a light stretch in your triceps. Press yourself back up, straighten your arms and repeat for 10 reps.

4. Dumbbell Curls

This exercise will help strengthen your biceps, which are the muscles in the front of your upper arms. Grab a set of light dumbbells - even a 2-pound set will work if that's all you have on hand at home - and stand with your feet shoulder-width apart. Keep your arms straight with a slight bend at the elbow, and lift them up towards your shoulders without moving them forward or back as you curl them up towards you chest. Squeeze your biceps at the top of the movement, and slowly bring them back to the starting position. Repeat for 8 to 10 reps.

5. Reverse Crunch

This exercise will help strengthen your core muscles, which are the ones in your abdomen and lower back. Lie on the floor with your knees bent up near your chest and feet flat on the ground. Place both hands behind your head or underneath your neck with elbows out (like you were going for an upside down push up). Lift yourself off of the ground by tightening in abs and pulling yourself up as if you were trying to touch your feet with your chest. Squeeze your abdominals as you exhale, and slowly lower yourself back down to the floor. Repeat for 10 reps.

6. One-Legged Dead Lift

This exercise will help strengthen your hamstrings and glutes, which are some of the largest muscles in the back of your legs. To do it, grab a barbell with a wide

grip near the ends of its handle (but not so wide that it is hard to hold). Stand up straight with your feet shoulder-width apart and knees facing forward so that the barbell is hanging in front of you. Slowly bend at the waist while keeping your back straight and pulling down on the barbell with both hands until you feel a stretch in your hamstrings.

Chapter 3: Cardio and Mind-Body Training

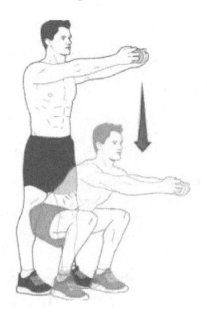

The best cardio workouts last about 45 to 60 minutes—and they can lead to a leaner body. That's how long it takes to get your heart rate up, burn calories and elevate the metabolism. That's also not what we're going for. Our goal here is to burn fat, which is why I have designed a set of 15-minute workouts that will help you access your fat stores and burn more fat after each workout. These workouts don't require the same amount of time from you because they aren't as intense as traditional cardio sessions that last an hour or more. But don't let that fool you—this isn't a light workout by any means. You will definitely feel them the next day because it takes a lot of work to burn calories and to build endurance. But the good thing is, you'll look forward to your workouts when they're over and you realize how much of a difference they are making in your life. This program will help you burn calories soon after each workout thanks to that calorie-burning effect called excess post-exercise oxygen consumption, or EPOC. You can think of EPOC as the afterburn effect, which makes it so that even after you are finished exercising, your body continues working for up to 24 hours after every workout session and burns more fat during that time. The only way to get this effect is to burn a lot of fat. The workouts in this program will help you do that. There are seven workout sessions in the program, and each one will last 15 minutes. I designed those short workouts to maximize your time and your results. They will help you burn calories and build endurance without being too intense or taking up too much time from your day. Each workout session uses a different cardio exercise so that you don't get bored from doing the same thing every day. Your muscles, joints and ligaments need rest in between exercises - especially if you are new to barbell training or resistance training in general. This program assumes that you are starting out with a basic understanding of how to lift weights, or that you have already gained enough control over your body and its movements to be able to complete the exercises safely. If you aren't sure if this program is right for you, talk with a certified trainer or fitness professional who can help you decide whether or not it is a good fit for your current fitness level.

To get the most out of this workout plan, do each session 2 or 3 times per week. You can do it every other day, but I would recommend spacing them out by at least two days so that your muscles have some time to repair themselves between training sessions. If you are just starting out, you might want to choose a lighter exercise session for days when you are doing your upper body workout. If you aren't sure which workout session is right for your fitness level, talk with a certified trainer or fitness professional who can help you decide.

1. Bodyweight Squats

This is a great way to warm up before your workout. It's not only good for building strength and increasing flexibility, it also burns calories. Stand with your feet shoulder-width apart and hold your arms out in front of you at shoulder height with palms facing down. Lean your weight back into your heels, and lower yourself towards the ground while flexing your knees to 90 degrees. Keep going until you feel a light stretch in your calves or thighs, then press back up and repeat for 50 reps.

2. Pushups

This is another great workout to do as a warm-up. Pushups are a compound exercise that work out your chest, abs and shoulders, and they also help strengthen your triceps and biceps. To do them, lie facedown with your hands spread out about shoulder-width apart underneath you. Lower yourself towards the ground until your chest nearly touches it while keeping your elbows at

90 degrees. Press yourself back up to the starting position by pushing with your arms, shoulders and chest. Repeat for 50 reps.

3. Lunge Jumps With Pushup

This is a bodyweight exercise that will definitely get you sweating! To do it, start in a standing position with feet shoulder-width apart and hands on hips. Step forward with one foot about two and a half feet out from your body, and bend both knees until you feel a light stretch in your thigh. Your back knee should be nearly touching the ground, but keep it just an inch off the ground without letting it touch. Press yourself back up to the starting position by pushing with your front leg muscles, then jump up as high as you can and land softly on the ground in the same position you were in when you started. Repeat for 15 reps on each leg.

4. Skaters

This is another compound exercise that will get your heart pumping! To do this exercise, stand with feet shoulder-width apart and arms out at your sides with palms facing forward. Jump up and down on your toes, and move your arms back and forth in a running motion while you jump. The faster you are moving your arms, the easier it will be to get your heart rate up. Repeat for 25 jumps.

5. Leg Lifts

This exercise is great for toning and strengthening your lower abdominal area! Start lying on the floor with legs together and arms at your sides with palms facing down. Raise both legs off the ground as high as you can by bringing in both the front and back sides of both legs. Squeeze those same muscles on the way back down to the starting position, then repeat for 15 reps.

6. Walking Lunges

This bodyweight exercise is one of my favourites - it exercises so many different muscles at once! Stand with your feet shoulder-width apart and arms out in front of you at shoulder height with palms facing down. Step forward with one foot about two and a half feet out from your body, and bend both knees until you feel a light stretch in your thigh. Your back knee should be nearly touching the ground, but keep it just an inch off the ground without letting it touch. Press yourself back up to the starting position by pushing with your front leg muscles, then jump up as high as you can and land softly on the ground in the same position you were in when you started. Step forward with your other leg, then repeat for 15 reps on each leg.

7. Burpees

This is another compound exercise that will get your heart pumping! Burpees are a full body exercise that burn a lot of calories and strengthen all of the major muscles in your body, including your arms, shoulders, back and chest. To do them, start standing up straight with feet shoulder-width apart and hands on hips or at shoulder height with palms facing down. Jump up as high as you can towards the ceiling by pushing from both legs and throwing both arms straight out in front of you. Press yourself back up to the starting position by bending at the knees and hips, then

immediately jump into the air again and repeat for 15 reps.

8. Side Knee Lifts

This is another exercise that is great for toning your lower abdominal area! Start lying on a side with one leg straight out in front of you and the other bent at a 90 degree angle with foot flat on the ground. The bottom foot can be flat or you can lift it off of the ground slightly. Lift you top knee as high as you can towards your chest while keeping your hips up, then lower it back down to the starting position. Repeat for 50 reps, then switch sides and repeat with your other leg.

9. Mountain Climbers

This is another full body exercise that will get your heart pumping! Start out in a push-up position with back straight and feet together. With one leg, step forward so that your knee comes up to your chest while you are still in the push-up position. When you bring your knee back down to the floor, switch legs and repeat on that side. Repeat for 15 reps, then switch sides and repeat with your other leg.

10. Plank Jumps

This bodyweight exercise is an excellent workout for strengthening both of your arms since the resistance comes from holding yourself up! To do it, lie face down with upper torso off of the floor so that you are resting on forearms and toes. Hold yourself up as long as you can, then jump up and land softly on the floor. Repeat for 15 jumps.

11. Plank Holds

This exercise will help strengthen your core muscles and keep your body toned! To do it, lie face down on the floor with legs together and arms at your sides with palms facing down. Raise both legs off the ground as high as you can by bringing in both the front and back sides of both legs without dropping either of your shoulders or hips to the floor while holding yourself up with forearms and toes. Hold that position as long as you can, then lower yourself back to the starting position by slowly lowering both

arms, feet and hips to the ground before repeating for 3 minutes.

Cardio Workouts are great because they get your heart rate up and help you stay focused during each exercise session. The key to success is to make sure you find a plan that will work for your body and your current fitness level. You should be able to push yourself each time you exercise, but you should also make sure that the exercises are challenging enough to allow room for progress when you return to that routine again. Only by pushing yourself will you see results, so find a workout plan that is right for you and start seeing changes today!

Cardio Workouts are great because they get your heart rate up and help you stay focused during each exercise session. The key to success is to make sure you find a plan that will work for your body and your current fitness level. You should be able to push yourself each time you exercise, but you should also make sure that the exercises are challenging enough to allow room for progress when you return to that routine again. Only by pushing yourself will you see results, so find a workout plan that is right for you and start seeing changes today!

This program is a perfect example of how getting in shape doesn't have to be hard or boring! If you currently don't have any workout routines, this plan has all of the tools and suggestions you need to get started on your path towards a healthier life.

Chapter 4: 15-Minute Training Plans

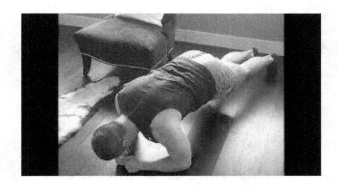

Cardio Workouts are great because they get your heart rate up and help you stay focused during each exercise session. The key to success is to make sure you find a plan that will work for your body and your current fitness level. You should be able to push yourself each time you exercise, but you should also make sure that the exercises are challenging enough to allow room for progress when you return to that routine again. Only by pushing yourself will you see results, so find a workout plan that is right for you and start seeing changes today! These 15-minute training plans can be used for aerobic workouts or resistance training. They are all great if you have little time in your day but want a quick, effective workout.

1. The 5-Minute Workout If you are really short on time and want to get an intense workout in, then this program is perfect for you. It's a great way to get your muscles pumping and to start sweating with just a few minutes of exercising!

2. The 10-Minute Workout This workout plan is easy and quick, yet still gets results! It can be used as a stand-alone workout plan or as extra cardio work after you have already performed a longer training session on another day. Many people find that it helps them lose weight and stay focused on exercise when they do this less intensive training after their long workouts are over for the week.

3. The 15-Minute Workout This full-body training program will get your heart pumping in just fifteen short minutes! It's a great way to get your body warmed up and ready for more intense workouts later in the week.

4. The 30-Minute Workout Many people find that they have time to exercise in the mornings before work, but if you have

trouble keeping yourself motivated in the mornings, then this program is for you! This routine is designed to be done right after waking up so that it doesn't interfere with your breakfast or morning routine.

5. 30-Minute Upper Body Workout Whether you are trying to impress the ladies or just want to look good shirtless, this workout plan will give you the muscles you're looking for in just thirty minutes! This program is perfect for everyone - men, women and even children.

6. The 30-Minute Full Body Workout This full body training program is great for building muscle and increasing endurance. It's a perfect training plan to help you get into shape after a long break from working out or if you want to train more intensely than usual.

7. The 30-Minute Lower Body Workout If you want to really build muscle in your biceps, quads and calves, then this is the training plan for you. It's a great way to train all of the muscles in your lower body if you are trying to improve your

overall strength or if you want to increase the muscle on a specific part of your body.

8. The 30-Minute Upper & Lower Body Workout This workout program is designed specifically for people who want to work on both their upper and lower body with equal intensity at the same time! It's a great training plan that will tone and strengthen your muscles while also working on mobility and endurance.

Full body program that uses both free weights and exercise machines to tone and strengthen your entire body. This workout plan is great for people who want to focus on building muscle or toning their entire body with just fifteen minutes of exercising each day. This training plan will get your heart pumping and help you burn fat all over your body! It's also great as a supplement to other training programs, so use it as an extra workout after you have already put in a longer training session. It's never too late to start becoming the best version of yourself!

This stand-alone workout plan is designed specifically for people who want to work on their upper body and nothing else. If you currently lift weights or do other exercises to build your muscles, then this workout plan can be added on after you have finished a longer training session that works on areas other than your arms, shoulders, chest and back. It's a great way to increase the intensity of your training sessions if you find yourself too tired or short on time for a longer workout later in the week. Use it alone or as an extra workout after you have completed a longer training routine on another day.

This bodyweight training program uses various muscles in your body to tone and strengthen your muscles. It's great for quick workouts that don't take too long but will still give you the results you are looking for! This program is also great for kids who want to keep their bodies healthy while they are growing up. This bodyweight training program is great for getting in shape without taking up your precious time! It's a great way to stay fit when you are travelling, working

late or if you just have very little time for exercising. It will help keep your muscles strong and improve your endurance while helping you burn fat all over your body.

Endurance is essential for staying healthy and strong throughout the years. If you want to train your body to be able to run fast and far, then this program is perfect for you! It's designed to be a long distance training plan that will help you run faster and farther than ever before by increasing your endurance. It's perfect for people who already have experience running or prefer not to use weight training programs. This program will help you tone and strengthen your muscles while also building up the muscles in your legs. The best way to improve the strength of your legs is by increasing the amount of weight that they are lifting, so this program does just that!

This high intensity interval training (HIIT) workout plan is great for people who want a quick workout with high intensity. Your heart rate will be elevated for the entire workout plan, so this is a great way to burn fat and keep yourself in shape! It's also perfect for people who want to increase the intensity of their workouts but don't have much time to work out. Remember that you should only do this workout 2-3 times a week, as it is intense and will take its toll on your body if you do it more often.

Chapter 5: The Top 10 Motivators to Work Out for 15 Minutes or Less

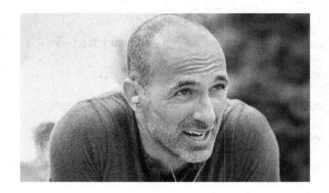

Are you looking for some motivation to get your workout on? If you need a little extra push to get up and start exercising, then look no further. This chapter will provide you with the motivation and tools you need to get moving today! Motivation plays an important part in your ability to stay fit and healthy, so make sure that you have the proper motivation before heading out into the world for a run or a workout at the gym. This chapter will also give you some great tips on how to stay motivated when working out can be hard. These are all great ways that top athletes use to keep themselves motivated on days when they think they can't go on. When you're looking for a little motivation,

remember that these athletes are regular people who use these techniques to push themselves harder. It may not work for everyone, but it's worth a shot! Here are the top ten motivators to get you started:

1. Exercise with Someone Who Keeps You Motivated Whether you are going to a class or working out alone at the gym, make sure you find someone who will keep you motivated throughout your workout. Working out with a friend can make workouts more enjoyable and will keep you pushing yourself until the very end.

2. Do Something You Love Sometimes exercising can be hard if it feels like a chore that doesn't make any sense to do in the first place. If you are looking for a way to make working out more fun, then try finding something you love to do that gets your heart racing. Maybe you like a certain sport, or maybe just jogging outside is what makes you happy. If there's something that makes your heart pump and your body move, then use it as a motivator to push yourself harder!

3. Set a Goal to Meet Sometimes it's easy to lose sight of why we're doing this in the first place. If you are looking for some motivation, then create a specific goal for yourself that will keep you on the right track towards success. If you want to lose weight, then keep that goal in mind every time you exercise and it will keep you focused on your success.

4. Plan a Specific Time for Working Out If you are looking for motivation, then the best way to stay motivated is to plan a specific time that you can work out. This is especially helpful if you have trouble staying motivated or getting up early in the morning. Even if it's just 5 minutes a day, planning specific times can help get your body moving even when you don't think you can.

5. Think About What You Could Do Without It Sometimes it's hard to understand what we have until we lose it altogether. If you are having trouble getting motivated, then think about what you would be missing if you weren't able to work out. What would your life be like if you hated going to the gym?

Would your clothes fit right? Would your health be in danger? Would you look physically different with all of that extra weight on your body?

6. See Yourself at a Specific Weight When working out, sometimes it's easy to forget how far you have come and what your goal is in the first place. If you see a great picture of yourself looking fit and healthy, then use it as motivation to keep going when things start getting tough. It will remind you of your original goal and keep you on the right track to success.

7. Listen to Motivating Music There are lots of ways to get motivated in the world today, and one of them is listening to music that makes you want to move! Music with a strong beat and energizing lyrics can really push you harder during your workout. Some people find it hard to get into a rhythm when exercising without music while others think it takes away from their workout, but no matter what, listening to specific songs can be great motivation when working out.

8. Focus on What You Have Already Achieved Working out is all about achieving as much as we possibly can. Sometimes it's easy to forget how far we have come with our workouts, but if you are having trouble getting motivated, then think about what you have already accomplished. Maybe you ran a mile this week or maybe your muscles look a little more toned. Think about everything that you have already done and use that as motivation to continue on the right track towards success.

9. Focus on What You Are Doing While Working Out Sometimes it can be hard to motivate yourself when working out because you don't feel like working out in the first place! If you are finding yourself lacking motivation, then try focusing on what your body is doing while exercising rather than focusing on actually doing the workout itself. This will help you stay focused and keep your motivation on the right track.

10. Use a Workout Buddy Having a workout buddy can be extremely helpful if you are looking for some extra motivation to get you through your workout plan. If you have someone to exercise with, then make sure that they are serious about their workouts so that they can push you harder! It may also help if they are trying to do the same thing as you – whether that is losing weight or getting stronger – than working out with them will be a great way to reach your goal faster than ever before.

Chapter 6: The 15-Minute Workout Log

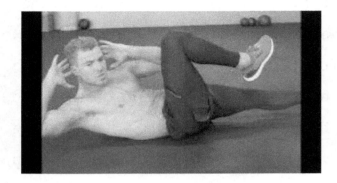

Keep track of your workouts with the workout log! This chapter will show you how to log your workouts for fifteen minutes or less. You will be able to keep track of your daily progress and create a custom workout plan that will keep you at a specific heart rate. This chapter will also give you some tips on how to make sure that your heart rate is right throughout each exercise. Depending on the workout program that you are using, it can be difficult to know exactly when to stop exercising during your training session. There are various ways to monitor this, but one of the best ways is using a heart rate monitor. It is most accurate if you have a heart rate monitor that works with your Smartphone, but it can also be used with free apps on your phone. This way, you can make sure that your heart stays in the right range and doesn't get too high or too low while working out. This is also great because it allows you to monitor your heart rate while running or exercising outside. If you plan on running, then make sure that your heart rate is monitored and stay in the correct heart rate zone. If you are looking for a quick way to monitor your heart rate, then you can always use a free app on your phone or hear rate monitor that is designed for high intensity workouts.

These are some of the best ways to keep track of your fitness:

1: The Basic Log This is probably one of the most common ways to track your workout. If you want something simple and easy to use, then this might be the best way for you. It's great because it's simple and it works! All you have to do is record basic information, such as the date and time, what you did during your workout, how long it took and maybe some additional notes about how it went. Record this in a notebook, on your computer or if you are using an app, then use that to log the information.

2: The Calorie Log If you are looking to lose weight, then this might be the log for you. This will help you keep track of your calories burned throughout the day and it will also tell you exactly how many calories you've burned during each workout session. This helps because it will keep track of everything for you and make sure that your fitness routine is working. It will also help to encourage you if things start getting tough because it will show how much progress you have made so far.

3: The Custom Log Depending on which fitness routine you are using, you might want to create a custom log. This way, you can keep track of everything that you should be doing and make sure that your body is getting what it needs. If there are certain exercises that you know your body needs, then make sure that those exercises are getting done! Use a spreadsheet or contact paper as a way to track your progress.

4: The Simple Log If you are looking for something simple and easy to use, then this might be the best choice for you. This will help keep track of some basic information and provide a little structure so that you know exactly how to keep track of your workouts. However, if you are using this log and you want more of a challenge, then try adding some extra exercises that you can do during your workout.

5: The Specific Log If you are looking for something simple and easy to use, but also want to keep track of your heart rate throughout the entire workout, then this might be the log for you. It has been designed specifically for workouts that last around fifteen minutes or less. All you have to do is follow the recommended heart rate zone that works best for your body and then record it throughout the workout. This way, you will know exactly what your heart rate should be at any given moment during the workout session.

6: The Workout Log Keeping track of your workouts is important whether you're training for a competition or just looking to get healthier and more fit. However, it can be a challenge to figure out what information you should be keeping track of and which information isn't necessary. This type of log will allow you to keep track of exactly how you are doing and how many calories you've burned during each workout session. It also keeps an accurate record of your heart rate zones so that you can make sure that your heart stays in the right range for the entire duration of the workout.

Chapter 7: The Equipment You Need

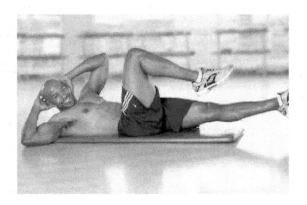

If you are going to be working out at home, then you will need a few pieces of equipment to really get the most out of your fitness routine. You don't have to have a lot of equipment in order to workout and be successful, but it would be ideal if you could find some good quality equipment that is easy for you to use. This chapter will show you the best types of equipment for using at home and how much each item costs.

The Best Equipment for Home Use

1: Two 5-pound dumbbells If you are just starting out and looking for something simple that won't cost much, then 5-pound dumbbells might be the right choice for you. These are usually the least expensive and can help you get in shape by using them for basic exercises.

If you are looking for something to work your arms and shoulders, then these will be a great choice.

2: Two or Three 10-pound dumbbells If you are looking for something stronger than 5-pound weights, then 10-pound weights might be a better option for you. These will help build your strength and endurance much faster and are also good for working out your arms and shoulders.

3: One 25-pound dumbbell If you are looking to start lifting heavier weights, then this might be the best choice for you. This is also a good weight for working out your shoulders and arms.

4: A 10-pound medicine ball If you are looking to add some variety to your weight lifting routine, then a medicine ball will be a great choice for you. These are great for working out your upper body and building strength in your core. They can also help you improve balance and stability if you throw them around while working out.

5: A foam roller Foam rollers are a relatively new piece of equipment that have come about over the last few years of fitness training. If you have never tried one, then they can help relieve pain in your muscles after exercising or running long distances.

6: A weighted jump rope If you want to get a good jump rope, then this might be the best choice for you. These ropes come in various weights, but they are great for increasing your cardio and building up endurance. They are also really fun to use!

7: A jump mat This is another great choice and will help you stay safe while doing basic exercises like sit-ups or push-ups. These mats can also help decrease the risk of injury while doing cardio workouts.

8: Resistance bands If you need something to work your legs out without stepping on a treadmill or run outside, then resistance bands might be the right choice for you. These come in various sizes and are great for targeting specific muscles.

Finding the Best Equipment for Home Use If you are looking to purchase any of these items, then look online at stores like Target or Amazon, or try a local sports equipment store. Make sure that the equipment is high quality and will last you a long time. They should also be easy to use and should be able to help you reach your workout goals in no time!

Chapter 8: The Healthiest Foods on Earth: Super foods to Fuel Your 15-Minute Workouts and Other Health Longer.

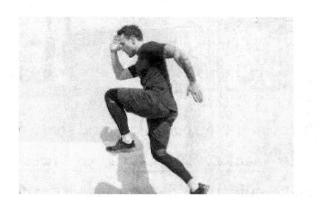

This is a list of some of the healthiest foods on earth, as well as what they can do for you. These are great to have in your fridge, so make sure that you grab something healthy to eat after a hard workout session.

7 Food Superstars for Healthy Hearts Heart disease is one of the most common causes of death in America, but there are ways to keep your heart healthy. One of the best ways to do this is by eating healthy foods. These are the healthiest foods that you can eat for your heart and some of them may surprise you.

1: Grapefruit This crispy fruit is full of nutrients and vitamins that are good for your heart and blood vessels. They also have a lot of potassium in them, which helps lower blood pressure and reduce risk of stroke. If you're feeling like your heart isn't getting enough attention, then grapefruit might be a great way to help!

2: Avocados Remember these from your favourite guacamole? They actually have a ton of health benefits because they are filled with omega-3 fatty acids, vitamin E, vitamin C and potassium. They are also good for preventing coronary heart disease and cardiac arrest.

3: Oatmeal It might be common knowledge that oatmeal is good for your diet, but did you know that it is also great for your heart? It is full of soluble fibber which can help lower cholesterol and blood sugar levels.

4: Herring If you were looking to eat something savoury, then this might be what you're looking for! Herring has omega-3 fatty acids which help to reduce cholesterol and triglyceride levels in the blood. These are also great if you have a hard time eating leafy greens or other vegetables because they can be added to almost any dish.

5: Salmon Salmon is another fish that is great for your heart. It is full of omega-3 fatty acids and vitamin D, which are both important for reducing the risk of heart disease. This fish also has enough Omega-6 Omega-3 fatty acids to help your body absorb more fat and prevent heart disease and high blood pressure.

6: Tomatoes Remember to eat the skin because it may not be as healthy as you think! These bad boys are low in calories, but high in lycopene and antioxidants. They also have lots of fibre to help keep you full longer and improve digestion.

7: Beans These are one of those healthy foods that you probably remember from your childhood. They are great for heart health because they have lots of fibre, protein and potassium in them. If you don't like black beans, then you can try out some pinto beans or kidney beans as a way to help your heart stay healthy.

The Best Foods for Your Heart If you want to be sure that your heart is staying strong and healthy, then consider adding some of these foods to your diet. Eating healthy gives your body what it needs to stay healthy and also avoids some of the diseases that plague people every day.

The Best Foods for Your Brain

3 Super Foods for Focused Thinking and Improved Memory

If you want to keep your mind sharp and your memory intact, then you need to make sure that you are eating healthy foods. This focuses on three foods that are great for maintaining focus while exercising or just trying to get through work. These super foods also improve memory and can help keep your mind sharp while giving you a fun boost of energy when you need it most.

1: Walnuts This is a great source of omega-3 fatty acids and antioxidants that help to protect your brain from age-related memory loss. These nuts also contain lots of vitamin E, which is great for learning and memory.

2: Avocado Peppers This might be one of the most delicious super foods out there, but did you know that it is also full of good fats that can improve memory? It has vitamin B6 in it as well, which helps regulate blood sugar levels.

3: Wild Blueberries Blueberries are one of the healthiest fruits on earth and they come packed with nutrients that are good for your brain. These berries are also full of vitamin C, which helps to reduce stress and improve focus. If you eat a handful of these berries before a workout or before work, then you will be giving your body and mind the boost that it needs.

The Best Foods for Your Brain If you want to exercise your mind as well as your body, then consider eating any of these super foods on a regular basis. Those who eat healthy live longer and tend to have fewer health issues than those who don't!

The Best Foods for Your Colon
3 Super Foods for Happy Digestion

Your digestive system is responsible for absorbing nutrients from all the food in your diet. It needs to be healthy to get all the nutrients that you need, but it can also be affected by stress and illness. This will teach you about three foods that are great for improving digestion and keeping your colon in good shape!

1: Broccoli This might be a familiar vegetable, but did you know that it is great for your colon? It has lots of fibre, potassium and vitamin C in it, which are all essential in keeping your digestive system moving the right way.

2: Parsley Did you know that parsley is actually healthy? It is full of antioxidants and fibre that can help prevent bad stomach problems like constipation or diarrhoea. These are great for people who experience bloating or indigestion regularly.

3: Beans Beans are one of the healthiest foods on earth and they are full of fibre that will help clean out your colon. They also have lots of protein in them, which helps to regulate your stomach and improve digestion.

The Best Foods for Your Colon If you want to stay regular and happy, then consider eating any of these super foods on a regular basis. If you regularly have problems with bloating or indigestion, then this can help you regulate your stomach and get rid of the bloated feeling.

Chapter 9: The 15-Minute Mind-Body Workout Plan for a Better Brain and a Calmer You

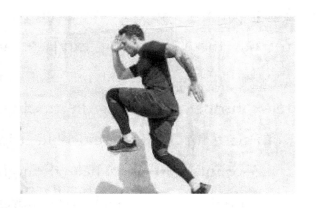

This is a sample workout plan that can be used for working on your brain or body. You should be able to do this at home with very little equipment and it only takes 15 minutes! Just get yourself ready and go over the plan to see how you can work out your body in just 15 minutes. This is easier than you think!

1. 2-3 Warm Up Exercises This will help loosen up your muscles before you do the rest of the workout. Try walking for 3 minutes and then stretch your arms, legs, back and shoulders before you attack the rest of your workout.

2. 3-4 Strength Exercises These exercises will help build up your muscles and start to burn calories. Do each exercise

for around 30 seconds and then take a short break before you move on to the next one.

3. 2-3 Cool Down Exercises If you are looking for something to cool down your body, then use the next few exercises to stretch out your muscles and get loose again. Try sitting down in a chair with your legs stretched out in front of you and lean back with one hand behind your head. This will help improve flexibility in your shoulders and hips.

4. 2-3 Stretching Exercises If you want to get even more flexible, then try three more stretches for your hips, legs and arms. Hold each stretch for around 30 seconds and then roll your shoulders and neck to loosen them.

5. 3-4 Breathing Exercises These breathing exercises are great for calming your mind and preparing you to finish the workout. They will also help regulate your heartbeat as well as boost energy levels. To do these exercises, breathing in through your nose for 3 counts and hold it in

for 3 counts. Slowly exhale for 6 counts before taking a deep breath again.

6. 2-3 Deep Breathing Exercises You should also try out some deep breathing exercises at the end of the workout to help you relax. Breathing in through your nose for 5 counts and slowly exhale for 10 counts. Repeat this 6 times to get rid of stress and relax.

7. 2-3 Meditation Exercises If you want something a little more challenging, then meditation exercises are a great way to finish the workout. Sit down with your back straight, close your eyes and focus on your breathing for two minutes. This will help keep you relaxed and focused before continuing on with the rest of your day.

8. 2-3 Cool Down Exercises If you want to stretch out your muscles after the workout, then be sure to do it using the next few exercises. Try sitting in a chair with your legs outstretched in front of you and lean back with one

hand behind your head. This will help improve flexibility in your hips and shoulders.

9. 3-4 Breathing Exercises You can also try out these breathing exercises at the end of the workout to help you relax further. Breathing in through your nose for 3 counts and hold it in for 3 counts. Slowly exhale through your mouth for 6 counts before taking a deep breath again.

Chapter 10: The 15-Minute Exercises You Can Do Anywhere

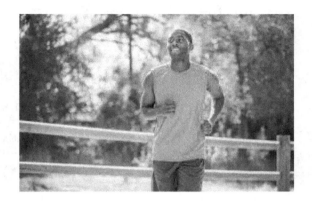

Did you know that you can do a workout without a gym? It's true! You can do it almost anywhere and with the right exercises, you can get in shape in less than 15 minutes. This is the best part of all because it doesn't matter where you are when your body needs to be exercised. Here are some of the best exercises that you can try out.

1. 2-3 Warm Up Exercises Warming up before your workout is one of the most important things that you need to do and it only takes about 5 minutes for this. You should start off by walking for 2 minutes and then stretch your arms, shoulders, legs and back for another minute. When you feel ready to move on, then you can jump right into the workout.

2. 3-4 Strength Exercises Pick 3 different exercises for your body and do each one for 1 minute before taking a break. You should try squats, lunges and pushups at first to work out your core as well as your legs. You can also try arm raises to work out your arms.

3. 3-4 Cool Down Exercises After you are done with the strength exercises, then use the next few minutes to cool down with some more stretching and breathing exercises. Try sitting in a chair with your legs extended in front of you and lean back while resting one hand behind your head.

4. 2-3 Stretching Exercises After you have cooled down, then be sure to do some more stretching for your arms, legs and shoulders. You should also roll your neck and shoulders to loosen them up. If you want to take the best care of your body, then you should try out these exercises so that you can get back in shape in a safe and effective way!

5. 2-3 Breathing Exercises These exercises are great for relaxing your body and helping it to stay calm throughout the day. To do them, breathe in through your nose for 5 counts before holding it in for 10 counts. Slowly exhale through your mouth for 8 counts before taking another deep breath. This helps to reduce stress and calm your body down.

6. 2-3 Deep Breathing Exercises This is one of the hardest parts of any workout, but it's important that you try them out! To do these exercises, breath in through your nose for 5 counts and slowly exhale through your mouth for 10 counts. Repeat this 6 times to help relax your body and mind.

7. 2-3 Meditation Exercises These are the most difficult exercises of all because they take a lot of focus to do correctly. If you want something more challenging, then sit in a chair with your back straight, close your eyes and focus on breathing for 2 minutes.

This will help keep you relaxed and focused whenever you need to be.

8. 3-4 Breathing Exercises You can also try out these breathing exercises at the end of your workout to help you relax. Breath in through your nose for 4 counts and hold it in for 5 counts. Slowly exhale through your mouth for 8 counts before taking a deep breath again.

9. 2-3 Cool Down Exercises If you want to stretch out your muscles, then use the next few minutes to try some basic stretching exercises for your shoulders, arms and legs. This will help stretch out any tight muscles from the workout as well as loosen up tight joints that make it hard to move around easily.

10. 2-3 Stretching Exercises If you want to do a little more, then try some more stretching exercises for your arms, legs and shoulders. You should also roll your neck and shoulders to loosen them up and improve flexibility.

Chapter 11: A New You in Just 15 Minutes.

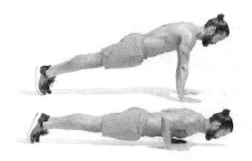

If you follow the workout plan in this book and eat healthy, then you will start to see a difference in your body and health. Your body will be happier, stronger and more flexible than ever before. This is how:

Eating Healthy You might have heard that eating healthy is the best way to improve your health, but do you know how it works? The food that we put into our bodies has to be able to digest easily so that we can absorb all of the nutrients that we need. If the food does not digest well, then it will go through your colon and get trapped there for a long time. This will cause your colon to become sluggish and fat deposits will build up behind the stool. Over time, your colon will get bigger and bigger because your body is not getting the nutrients that it needs. Your digestive system will eventually get blocked because it can no longer push the stool through your colon and out of your body. If you constantly eat foods that are hard to digest, then you will have to deal with serious lifestyle issues in the future. This is why you need to change your diet and start eating more vegetables and fruits instead of processed foods. You will also want to stop drinking soda or alcohol if you currently do. These drinks are full of sugar, which is hard for your body to absorb if you don't have enough fibre in your diet. Your digestive system needs fibres so that it can get rid of the unabsorbed food. If you are trying to lose weight, then focus on eating more vegetables and fruits. This will help you to get rid of excess water and boost your metabolism at the same time. You should also avoid fried foods because they are high in fat as well as saturated fats that will stick to the walls of your colon. You need to avoid this because it will make your body start to swell up and cause digestive problems like constipation, bloating or diarrhoea. Fiber is also very important for keeping a healthy digestive system and you can get it by eating lots of green leafy vegetables, oatmeal, oat bran, wheat bran and whole grains. Over time, you will see a huge difference in your digestive health and you should start to have much less constipation and bloating. Your body will no longer hold onto excess water or get impacted by extra pounds. You can also add some probiotic yogurt into your diet because it contains good bacteria that helps break down food so that it can be digested. This is very helpful for those that have digestive issues like diarrhoea because the good bacteria restores balance to their intestines after being sick or drinking certain beverages.

3-4 Minutes of Exercise Doing a few minutes of exercise every day will improve the way that your body moves. You will start to feel stronger, more flexible and much more relaxed. In fact, it only takes around 3 minutes of exercise to realize some of the health benefits which is why you should add 15 minutes into your busy schedule every day. Since you can do this in your own home or office, there are no excuses not to do it! When it comes to moving your body around, then try out some squats with weights and lunges. You should also try going for a walk around the block or even running up and down flights of stairs if you have the time. If you want to get even more movement in your body, then you should try out some yoga poses every day. You can do the sun salutation stretch or do some of the simpler moves like downward facing dog or child's pose.

3-4 Minutes of Breathing Exercises It is also important that you take the time to focus on breathing exercises that will help you to calm down and relax. You should try three different breathing exercises every day for at least 3 minutes each. Try out the diaphragmatic breath, corpse pose and box breathing exercise so that you can clear your mind and relax your body.

3-4 Minutes of Deep Breathing Exercises The most important thing that you can do is to practice deep breathing every day for a few minutes. This will help you to relax and calm down when you are feeling stressed or anxious. You should practice breathing exercises by sitting in a chair with your back straight and then breathe in through your nose for 5 counts before slowly exhaling through your mouth for 10 counts. Repeat this 6 times so that you can start to clear your mind and relax.

2-3 Minutes of Meditation Exercises If you want something that is a little more challenging, then focus on practicing meditation exercises every day for 2 to 3 minutes. This will help you to feel happy and relaxed for the rest of your day. You should sit somewhere comfortable with your back straight before closing your eyes and focusing on breathing for 2 minutes. This is a great way to get in a relaxed state and focus on the good things in your life as well as forget about everything else!

The Benefits Of Working Out In A Group

If you are trying to lose weight or get into shape, then you might be wondering whether it's better to do these things alone or with a group of friends. In fact, you can do both because each method has its own advantages and disadvantages. Here are some reasons as to why you might want to join a group in the future.

3-4 Reasons To Work Out In A Group

1. Accountability When you work out in a group, then it is easy to get distracted or start talking about other things that are going on in your life. This is why it's important for everyone to hold each other accountable so that they can be sure that the workout will happen as planned and nothing else will come up. When everyone is working out together, then no one wants to let the other people down by not being there or doing exercises incorrectly.

2. Motivation If you are suffering from motivation issues, then you should join a

group so that you can enjoy the fun of working out with your friends.

3. Healthy Competition Working out in a group will also help you to have healthy competition to keep your body motivated and moving in the right way. You should always expect to get the best results if you are working out with other people because this will encourage everyone to stay on track. It's important for everyone to keep each other accountable so that everyone succeeds together and it's not just one person that gets healthier while others go back to eating unhealthy foods or giving up on their goals.

4 Things To Do When Joining A Group

a. Try Out Different Workout Classes There are so many workout classes available for you to choose from, so it can be hard to know where to start. Luckily, you can try out different classes until you find one that matches your fitness level and goals. You should try out a class that is something new to you every few weeks so that you get the most benefits possible.

b. Check Your Level Of Skill If the rules of the class are too hard for you, then talk to your instructor about working at a different skill level or coming back again when your skills have improved. It's a terrible feeling to attend a high-level class when you are not ready to do the exercises yet, so talk to the instructor if you have any skill or ability issues.

c. Get To Know The Skill Of Other People One of the most important things that you can do is work out with other people that are at your skill level so that you can encourage each other to stay motivated and get better results over time. You should also talk to the others about what they like most about working out in a group and how they enjoy motivating each other on social media.

d. Workout With Other People For Accountability Having someone to work out with for accountability is very important and you should definitely invite your friends to join you as well. If they already work out, then it will be easy to go at the same time and do the same exercises. You can even take turns encouraging each other as you workout so that no one gets distracted by their surroundings or weakens when they are having a bad time.

3-4 Things To Avoid When Working Out in a Group

1. Obsessing Over Weight If you are truly working out with other people for motivation, then you should know that they are focused on their own results more than yours. If they want to lose weight, then they will follow their own program and it might be different from your workout plan so don't let this bother you. You can check out the same workout plan that your friend is following so that you push each other to stay accountable.

2. Spreading Bad Energy If you can't help but be negative about your workout or results, then don't bother joining a group. You will only end up spreading bad energy to others and they will lose faith in their fitness program.

3. Not Staying Safe If you are trying to work out in a group, then it's important to make sure that everyone is staying

safe at all times throughout the exercises so that no one gets injured. If you see that someone is doing something wrong, then point it out and see if they can correct their form so that they don't get hurt.

4. Not Getting Results You should also be aware that it might be a little harder to get results when you are working out in a group because you aren't sure what might affect your results. It's important for everyone to follow the same workout schedule so that everyone gets the results that they want over time.

The Benefits Of Yoga In a Mat

Yoga in a mat is a great exercise to try out because it will help you to have more flexibility, a stronger core and better balance. You should add this exercise to your workout schedule if you are looking for something new and low impact so that you can get the best results possible. To do this, follow these instructions.

1. Sitting Position The first step is to sit down on a soft mat with your legs crossed and your hands in your lap. You

want to either have the palms facing up or the fingers pointing toward the top of your head before you begin breathing exercises.

2. Breathing Exercises Next, you need to focus on your breathing by doing a breathing exercise for 3-4 minutes. You should breathe in for 5 counts before exhaling for 10 counts. You can practice this note breathing exercise for about 6 times to start feeling more relaxed and calm.

3. Lying Position Next, you need to lie down on your back before taking the time to focus on your breathing for 2 minutes. You should close your eyes and focus on breathing in for 5 counts before breathing out for 10 counts. This is a great way to get in a relaxed state and think about the things that are making you happy.

4. Sitting Position You can sit up after a few minutes and take the time to repeat the process once again if you want something more challenging or if you feel like being active.

5. Balancing Pose The next step is to stand up while you are holding a balancing pose for at least 3 minutes. You can do the tree pose, half moon, or warrior 1 pose to get in better shape and have a stronger core. You will feel much more flexible when you are done with this exercise and you should focus on getting a good stretch in your legs and back.

6. Standing Position Next, you should stand up while focusing on moving your body for another 2 minutes. While holding this position, you want to move around as much as possible so that you start burning fat from different areas of your body.

Conclusion

There are so many great exercises that you can do when working out in a group that can have an amazing impact on your life. You should definitely try these out because they are all exercises that someone else has already done and loved. If you want to get the best results possible, then focus on eating a healthy diet and exercising consistently. If you want extra motivation, then join a group and get better goals with friends! It's important for everyone to move their body and create new habits every day so that they can get healthier over time.

There are so many fun and interesting exercises that you can do when working out in a group, so it's important for everyone to try these out today. Who knows, you might even get the best results possible because of the people around you! It is also important to practice deep breathing every day for a few minutes so that you can calm down and relax your body when you are feeling anxious. This might be the most crucial part of working out in a group because it will get easier as time goes on. If you start focusing on your breathing every day, then it will only get easier for everyone who is living life with anxiety.

The 15-Day Women's Health Book of 15-Minute Workouts

By

Lil Ron

Table of Contents

Introduction

The 15-Day Fast Track to the Core Program is exactly that...a program that walks you step by step through a 15-minute workout template designed to take your body from a fat-storing machine into a lean, mean, calorie burning machine. OK, so you don't burn calories while sleeping or when you're sitting at your desk, but when you are exercising vigorously like in the 15-Minute Workout, you torch calories and fat at an accelerated rate. The program is designed to get the most out of each workout session by working every muscle group with tri-sets and supersets. The tri-sets and supersets are done so that you are constantly changing the angle of your muscles and joints. This keeps the workout from getting tedious and monotonous. It also increases your metabolism, thus preventing you from getting bored with the workouts.

This program is also designed to be as easy as possible in regard to equipment. I have tried my best to build a program that requires no equipment at all, or if you do have equipment, it should be simple and easy to get your hands on if you don't already own it. The only equipment you need is a set of dumbbells, though I do highly suggest you use a core stabilization ball and a resistance band. You can go to any department store and pick up these items, or if you are like me, your local grocery store has these readily available. The way I look at it is that if they sell it in the grocery store, then it must be pretty good for me! Now before we get into the program itself, I want to give you some tips on what to do with your day between workout sessions. We're not going to make our workouts longer but we will make them more productive by adding just two minutes of cardio work between the warm-up and cool-down period. This will help you burn more fat and calories throughout the day in between your workout sessions. How do I know what to do? Well, a lot of the things I have learned about working out is by studying bodybuilders. Bodybuilders aren't just people who want to be big and bulky...they also must have an incredible degree of muscular definition. The reason for this is that they are judged by how ripped their muscles are as well as how big they are when it comes to competitions such as the Mr. and Miss shows or Mr. Olympia! Bodybuilders know that if you wanted to win, you needed every muscle fibre in your body working together and functioning at its maximum capacity all the time. The only way you can do this is by having some sort of cardiovascular training done daily.

Chapter 1: What is the 15-Minute workouts?

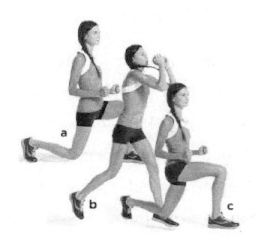

Work Smarter, Not Harder

Every second counts during your busy day—which is why you need a workout program that doesn't take up any of your precious minutes. So we asked our Men's Health Personal Trainer of the Year, Rachel Cosgrove, co-owner of Results Fitness in California and one of the country's top trainers, to create a fast workout routine for women. This 15-day plan will get you looking and feeling better fast.

Each day's workout targets a specific body part and burns about 400 calories. That's an extra 400 calories burned each day, just like that. And, since you're only doing 15 minutes at a time, you can squeeze in these workouts anytime—no

excuses! This plan is designed to be easy to follow at home or at the gym. You'll do seven supersets—a superset is when you alternate one set of an exercise with one set of another, back and forth without resting in between. The only rest you get is when it says REST (about a minute). Cosgrove will show you how it works in the video above.

Targeted Training for Busy Women

Each day's workout targets a specific body part with the goal of burning 400 calories. Example: If you do the plan on Monday and Wednesday, your week will be broken down as such: Monday—legs day and upper back day; Wednesday—arms and abs. This allows you to target your hard-to-tone trouble spots in just 15 minutes a day! The workouts are designed to be performed at home or at the gym. You'll do seven supersets—a superset is when you alternate one set of an exercise with one set of another, back and forth without resting in between.

A Healthier Lifestyle

Adding more exercise to your life can only benefit you, provided you exercise safely as discussed in more detail in the next chapter. However, if you are working out to lose weight in addition to becoming more physically fit, you will need to make changes to your diet as well.

The 15-Minute Body Fix will work best when accompanied by these changes. Observing portion sizes, choosing foods that are more nutritious, and limiting sugar, starch and alcohol will improve your health and the effectiveness of your workout.

Be aware, it's not necessary to change radically all aspects of your life at once. In fact, this can sabotage your plans before you really get started by overwhelming your system. Add elements of the 15-Minute Body Fix gradually to your life, and continue adding consistently until you are meeting your final goal.

All You Need Is You

A common complaint about beginning a fitness routine is expense: extensive equipment and videos to buy, or a pricey gym membership. All the workouts in the 15-Minute Body Fix are specifically chose to require little more equipment than your body weight.

Body weight workouts are designed to use your own weight instead of a dumbbell. These kinds of exercises place your body in what is called a disadvantaged position, requiring more strength to make the move. Pushups are the most famous of these exercises, but there are many more. These workouts also usually require the use of several muscle groups, so even if they are zone targeted, you will still continue to strengthen your other parts.

If any other equipment is involved, it will be a common household item, like a towel or a chair. You may also need to use a wall stabilize yourself. You will need a timer. However, a common kitchen timer will do, as will the stopwatch function on most cell phones. No fancy fitness equipment is needed for the 15-Minute Body Fix.

Chapter 2: The Science of Leanness

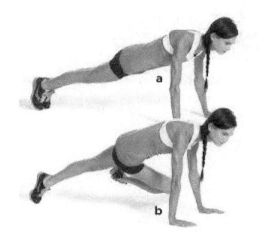

This is the most important chapter in the book. This chapter will teach you everything you need to know about how the human body burns fat and how you can rev up your metabolism so it's operating at its maximum efficiency even if you're not working out. I will also be covering a condition called insulin resistance which is a condition that slows down your metabolism and makes it harder for your body to burn fat. The good news is that insulin resistance is preventable by making small changes in everyday life. It's not something you just have to live with. You will find that in this program, the majority of your workouts focus around the muscles in the core area. The reason for this is because the core is considered to be one

of the most important areas for increasing calorie burning. I will also be teaching you how to rev up your metabolism with some simple but very effective exercises. To top it off, I'm also going to teach you about what and when to eat so that you can get all of the fat-burning benefits possible out of your diet plan!

Leanness Is NOT a Four-Letter Word

We have to change the way we look at fat and leanness in the modern day. The fitness world has made us think that being "fat" is something to be ashamed of and that putting on lean muscle is something that you have to work forever for. I'm here to tell you that this is simply not true! It's not true because all of us have fat on our bodies. We need fat to survive! It is true that our bodies can become much healthier if we have more lean muscle on our bodies and less fat but that's not the key. The key is getting leaner while preserving as much muscle tissue as possible. There are some people out there who believe that it's easier to lose weight by burning off as much of the muscle tissue as possible while you're going on a diet. The reason some people think this way is because they are always hungry and they feel lethargic. This is a complete lie! The easiest way to lose weight and keep your muscles intact is to consume just enough nutrients so you don't lose any muscle mass while losing body fat. If you consume an extreme amount of lean protein and just the right amount of carbohydrates, your body will enter a state called ketosis which is a state in which your body burns fat for energy instead of carbohydrates. The only time that carbs are burned is during intense exercise like sprinting. This mean that if you're at a standstill, your body is going to burn fat for energy instead of carbs. Keep in mind that this approach to getting leaner has to be done with long-term consistency. You cannot do this program once every two months and expect to see good results. You can only get the good results by making small changes to your daily life and doing it consistently over time. The worst thing that you can do is to try this program for 3 days and then quit. If you do that, all the time and money that you spent on your supplements will have been a waste. Over the next few sections, I'm going to teach you everything that I have learned over the past 12 years about losing fat while keeping muscle.

Diet

I would like to say it straight out the gate…"There is no quick fix diet!" There are some people who may lose fat quickly but those people are not eating healthy either. Just because you aren't hungry doesn't mean it isn't hurting your body. You will not get the best results with those crazy 3 day diets that you see on TV. Also, if there was a quick fix to losing fat, I could be gone by now. I would have already made my millions and wouldn't be writing these messages to you. There is no magic diet pill or potion that will make it easy for you to lose fat. The old adage "you can't out train a bad diet" cannot be put any more accurately than it is in this sentence. A good diet plays a significant role in getting leaner or building muscle because it is used as the source for your energy (calories) for your body to burn off of. If you don't have the proper nutrients coming in from your diet, your body is going to be forced to tap into muscles and fat tissue for energy. So having a good diet is a must for everyone, no matter what his or her goals may be.

Dieting Tips

1) Cut your portions- The easiest way to start decreasing the amount of calories that you are taking in is to simply cut your portion sizes down. Most people tend to eat overly large portions that main reason being that people cannot deal with having food go away on their plates. If you take in a large portion and finish it all, you feel accomplished. If the food that you ate was low calorie, then there shouldn't be anything to feel accomplished about. So I suggest taking your regular plate of food and half the size so that you're consuming less calories at each sitting. After the first week or two, get another plate of half the size and half with your original sized plate which will now be your medium sized plate. This will help you get into a routine of eating smaller portions by simply changing out your plates.

2) Eat more often- With the first tip, we want to start becoming in tune with our body's natural hunger signals. We can do this by simply eating more often. I suggest eating 4 meals a day, and 2 snacks. How you eat is not important as long as you are eating smaller portions and getting enough nutrients each day. As I will discuss in my nutrition plan, your meals should consist of a lean protein, fibre filled carbohydrate and a low glycemic index (low sugar) carbohydrate. This is just the basic outline for eating. As we get into the plan in the next few sections, I am going to tell you exactly what to eat for each meal.

3) Avoid sweeteners- Many people turn to sweeteners in order to cut calories from their diet and still have dessert. These sweeteners are usually found in desserts and beverages like soda or juice with little or no real nutritional value. These types of foods will sabotage your efforts because you will simply fill up on

them while not getting enough nutrients in your body. The best thing to do is avoid these types of foods all together. This may sound like it's impossible but if you just put in a little extra effort into planning your meals ahead of time, you will find that it's really not that hard and you will actually be able to enjoy more variety in your diet. I'm not suggesting that you have to cut out desserts for the rest of your life but what I am saying is that if you are trying to get leaner, then it doesn't make any sense at all to eat something that is going to sabotage your efforts.

4) Avoid Sodium- You may have heard this before...but sodium makes us retain water. If you are retaining water, it makes it look like you're not losing fat because your muscles are not as defined as they could be. So this is another area where you need to cut corners. Salt your food sparingly and find a low sodium sports drink or water if you are out and about. If you don't have time to prepare your own meals, try finding restaurants that serve mainly seafood or eat at home. It's much easier for them to control their

sodium levels than other types of restaurants.

5) Take your vitamins- Many times, when people go on a diet, they tend to forget about their vitamins and multivitamins. You should always take them even if you are eating a healthy diet. Vitamins and minerals are what make up muscles so without them, you will be losing weight from your muscles instead of fat. A fat loss and muscle building supplement is also a good option for you to use if you just aren't getting enough nutrients in your body each day (I will discuss this in my nutrition plan).

6) Keep Hydrated- I'm sure you've heard this many times but it's important so I'll say it again...Keep Hydrated! You should shoot for at least 8 glasses of water a day. Most people get all of their water from drinks like soda or juice which are just sugar water with no nutritional value what so ever.

7) Get Enough Sleep- I have already discussed how important sleep is in making muscle gains but another big

reason why it's important is because your metabolism is highest when you're sleeping. This means that you should be getting enough sleep each night. If you're only sleeping 5 hours per night, then try to get more by either going to bed earlier or waking up later in the morning.

Chapter 3: How to Maximize Post-Workout Recovery so You Can Train Harder and Recover Faster.

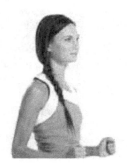

If you want to build a lean and muscular body, you have to train hard and often. Training hard is one thing if you can recover quickly, but if your muscles have a difficult time recovering after a heavy weight training session then all your hard work will be for nothing.

The goal of this chapter is to show you exactly what foods and supplements you can use to help your body recover fast from exercise.

1) Eat smart before going to bed- Try eating more the night before so that you wake up with an empty stomach (don't eat within 3 hours of going to sleep). Make sure your last meal before bed consists of mostly protein. This will help your body repair and recover from weight training while you sleep.

2) Sleep long enough- Not getting enough sleep is the main reason why people can't recover from exercise, because you body needs rest and recuperation. The average person should get between 7-9 hours of sleep per night.

3) Eat protein every 3-4 hours while awake- If you wake up at 6am, try eating a snack that consists of protein like a piece or two of chicken or drink whey protein (depending on your schedule). Then, eat a main meal that consists of a protein source like steak or chicken with a carbohydrate source. Then, have another snack that consists of protein like whey protein or a piece of deli turkey an hour or so after you eat your meal. Then, have another meal an hour after you have your snack and then eat dinner quite late at night (this way you will wake up with an empty stomach). Also, make sure to drink plenty of water to stay hydrated. If you are unable to eat every 3-4 hours while awake then take some type of protein supplement that uses slow-digesting proteins for long lasting amino acid delivery (whey is fast-digesting, casein is slow-digesting).

4) Take supplements- I would recommend taking some type of protein supplement before, during, and after exercise. You can use whey protein, casein protein, milk proteins (such as Optimum Nutrition 100% Whey Gold Standard), etc. I would also recommend using a multivitamin every day as well as 6-8 grams of BCAA's before and after exercise (I take Optimum Nutrition Amino Energy due to the fact that it contains creatine monohydrate). I recommend using creatine monohydrate because it has been proven to increase strength and lean muscle tissue over a period of time when taken consistently.

5) Eat regularly- Eating many small meals throughout the day is better for recovery than eating a few big meals.

6) Eat more fruits and vegetables- Fruits and vegetables contain important micronutrients that are important for recovery. Also, fruits and vegetables contain carbohydrates which you can absorb quickly to replenish muscle glycogen stores.

7) Eat healthy fats- Healthy fats such as olive oil, coconut oil, flaxseed oil, avocados, nuts, etc. help your body absorb the fat soluble vitamins A,D, E and K from the foods you eat.

8) Drink milk- Milk contains both slow-digesting proteins (casein) and fast-digesting proteins (whey). This makes milk a great post workout supplement.

9) Drink alcohol moderately- Drinking a glass of red wine daily has been shown to improve recovery from exercise.

10) Drink coffee- Research has shown that the amino acid L-Carnitine is found in higher levels in people who drink coffee compared to people who don't drink it. This is important because L-Carnitine helps transport fatty acids into the mitochondria of muscle cells so that they can be used as fuel for energy. The more fatty acids you can get into your mitochondria, the more fat you will burn throughout the day. Also, caffeine in coffee stimulates your central nervous system to make it easy for you to wake up and become highly alert.

Maximizing Post-Workout Recovery

Here is the list of foods and supplements that will help maximize post workout recovery:

1. Lean meats like chicken, turkey, and beef as well as fish

2. Eggs

3. Plant based protein powders

4. Whole milk

5. Whey protein powders (fast absorbing)

6. Casein protein powders (slow absorbing)

7. Multivitamins- Look for ones that contain calcium, magnesium, zinc, B vitamins, vitamin D3 (cholecalciferol), etc…

8. BCAA supplements- Drink these before and after training.

9. Creatine monohydrate

10. Caffeine from coffee or green tea

11. Fruits and vegetables

12. Healthy fats like olive oil, avocados, nuts, fatty fish (e.g., salmon), etc...

13. Milk- Consume this right after you train because it has both fast-digesting whey protein as well as slow-digesting casein protein in it (whey is fast digesting; casein is slow digesting).

14. Alcohol in moderation (e.g., 1 glass of red wine a day) has been shown to improve recovery from exercise .

Chapter 4: The Science of Muscular Strength

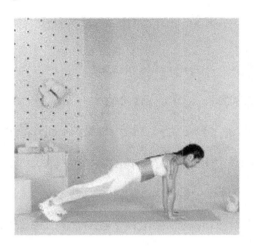

This chapter will teach you everything you need to know about building muscle. I'm not going to be teaching you how to do hundreds of different exercises. Instead, I'm going to be teaching you the most effective compound exercises (multi-joint) for each body part in terms of developing overall strength and increasing lean muscle mass. You will notice that there is a lot of attention paid towards your core muscles. Your core muscles are considered to be the most important muscle group in your body because they play a significant role in stabilizing your spine and increasing calorie burning. I will also be teaching you the different types of muscle fibres and how they help your body in everyday activities. Understanding how muscles work will help you to know what you need to do in order to build strength and muscle.

Muscular Strength and Development Facts

1) There are 2 types of muscle fibres found in our bodies. These are known as Type 1 and Type 2 muscle fibres. There is a simple way to remember them...Type 1 is called Slow twitch and Type 2 is called Fast Twitch. Slow twitch or Type 1 is designed for endurance, whereas fast Twitch or Type 2's main function is power. Slow twitch fibres burn more calories than fast twitch fibres which make them the best choice for your body when it comes to losing fat while preserving as much muscle as possible.

2) In order to build strength and aesthetics, you need to focus on compound exercises that work the major muscle groups of your body. Compound exercises are multijoint exercises (exercises that involve more than one major body part) that use large, powerful movements in order to help your body

develop overall strength. These are going to be the exercises that I will be focusing on for you over the next few chapters.

3) Whenever you feel fatigued during an exercise, it is usually a sign that you should stop the exercise and not push through with prolonged muscle failure. Prolonged muscle failure can cause your muscles to have delayed onset muscle soreness (DOMS) as well as take longer for your muscles to repair and rebuild themselves.

4) In order to build strength and muscle, you must eat enough calories and protein. Calories are the basic building blocks of energy needed for your muscles to repair themselves after an intense workout. Protein not only builds your muscles but it also helps them retain water which gives you a pumped look. I will discuss all of these nutrients as we get into my nutrition plan later on in this book.

5) Although I said that slow twitch fibres are more efficient for burning calories, they do not have the ability to explode or generate as much power as fast twitch

fibres can. This is why you need to use both types of exercises in order to develop strength and aesthetics (looks).

How The Body Creates Muscle

The task of strength and muscle development can be very complicated. I'm not going to get into the details of it, but I will give you a brief overview of what is happening during a typical muscle building process.

As we begin to lift heavy weights, two important reactions take place in the body. The first is that the brain releases a chemical known as adrenaline (epinephrine). Adrenaline speeds up the heart rate and makes more blood available for muscular contraction. This reaction increases muscular strength which is needed as your body begins to lift heavier weights. This reaction occurs for only a short period of time in order to maximize your ability to lift while not overworking your body.

The second reaction, which can last up to 48 hours after a rigorous workout session, is when your body releases growth hormone (GH). During this time,

GH stimulates the muscles to repair themselves as quickly as possible. This allows your body to build more muscle for future workouts. GH is also responsible for the burning sensation you feel 24-48 hours later.

In order to develop strength and increase lean muscle mass, you need to keep challenging your body by upping the intensity of your workouts. Your body will adapt within 3-4 weeks if you are training properly and doing more than just lifting light weights with poor form. You must keep your brain thinking that you're not capable of handling the amount of weight you are lifting if you want to continue to make progress.

Chapter 5: How to Build Lean Muscle (and Raise Your Metabolism)

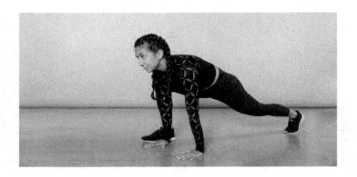

This chapter will be all about developing lean muscle mass. I will be discussing the six steps to building muscle and the type of equipment you should be using for each step. I will also give you a sample workout schedule to follow at the end. The first step to building muscle is stretching which I will discuss in this chapter as well.

I'm going to start by talking about how important it is for your muscles to stretch before and after every workout you do (this includes stretching your core). The main reason why it's important is because if you stretch the muscles, tendons and ligaments before a workout, then they are much more apt to being stretched during the workout as well. If you stretch before a workout, then your body will be much more flexible and

better capable of handling the stress of your weight training. Lifting weights puts a lot of pressure on the muscles that you are exercising. If you don't stretch before your workout, then the pressure on those muscles can cause them to tighten up and become very stiff which can result in muscle strains. I'm sure you know what this feels like from either experience or just seeing someone else with a muscle pull while working out. This is also known as delayed onset muscle soreness (DOMS) which I will discuss later on.

Understand that all of your workouts should be done in a progressive manner which means that each workout gets more intense than the last and that the weight you are using increases every week. There are six steps to developing lean muscle mass. These steps include: stretching, dynamic flexibility, active flexibility, traditional strength training, pre-exhaustion and super sets. Here they are in more detail:

1) Stretching- Before doing any kind of weight training or flexibility exercises,

you need to stretch for at least 10 minutes or until you feel completely stretched out. When doing this stretch routine, make sure to hold each stretch for 15 seconds before moving on to the next one (I'll discuss how to do each stretch later).

Stretching will do two things for you. First of all, it will improve your flexibility which is needed in order to perform some of the exercises I'll be teaching you. Secondly, it will help to keep your muscles from becoming tight which can result from being under too much stress while weight training (I explained how this works in the "Building Lean Mass" chapter).

2) Dynamic Flexibility- Dynamic flexibility is very similar to static stretching except that dynamic flexibility incorporates movement into the stretch so that you are actually moving through your range of motion. This type of stretching should also be done before your weight training workouts as well. The best way to do this is to start by loosening up your muscles and then move through your range of motion as you would when doing the actual exercise. I'll demonstrate this in more detail later on.

3) Active Flexibility- Active flexibility is basically doing the opposite of static stretching. Instead of holding a stretch for 15 seconds, you're going to hold it for 15 seconds or however long you can before your muscles begin to tighten back up and then contract yourself for 15 seconds (this applies when doing crunches or sit ups). This type of stretching should also be done before each workout session, especially lower body days.

4) Traditional Strength Training- This is what most people think of when they hear the words "weight training". This is where you use heavy weights and perform an exercise in a controlled manner in order to develop the strength of that particular muscle. You should use between 3-5 sets per exercise and do 4-6 repetitions for each set. When you are doing these exercises, don't just lift the weight up and down without any

control. You should be using your muscles to move the weight up and down. If you are just moving sluggishly through your range of motion then it means that you aren't getting a good workout.

5) Pre-Exhaust Training- Here you will be doing a set of an exercise for one particular muscle group and then immediately (with no rest in between) doing a set of an exercise that works the same muscle group but with a different range of motion. This is considered to be one superset. This is another way to challenge your body so that it continually adapts to the stress you are putting on it.

6) Super Sets- Here you will be doing two exercises for the same muscle group without any rest in between them. You should do each super set for 3 sets per exercise and 6 repetitions per set (I'll explain how to choose the right amount weight later).

Sample Workout Schedule

I am going to give you a sample workout schedule that you can try. This is a six day per week split routine and will involve several strength training exercises as well as active flexibility, dynamic flexibility and stretching for each muscle group. The first four days will be for training your upper body and the last two days will be for your lower body. It's important that you change up the order of these workouts every other week at least so that your body doesn't adapt to the workout routine repetition. Before each workout, warm up for 10-15 minutes by either doing some cardio or jogging in place (I will discuss warming up in more detail later on).

This schedule should be used as an example for you to follow and not as a "set in stone" plan. You need to change it up each time to make sure your body doesn't adapt to the same workout routine.

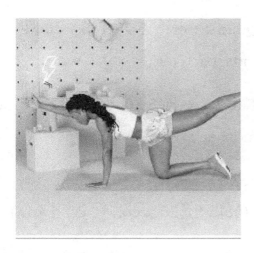

Day 1: Chest/Triceps (Rest Day)

A. Barbell Bench Press 3 x 8-12 reps

B. Cable Crossover 2 x 15-20 reps

C. Chest Stretch 5-10 reps (hold for 15 seconds)

D. Triceps Stretch (active flexibility) 5-10 reps (hold for 15 seconds)

E. Triceps Stretch (static flexibility) 10-15 reps

F. Clasping Triceps Stretch 10-15 reps

G. Clasping Rear Delt Stretch 10-15 reps

H. Chest Stretch 5-10 reps (hold for 15 seconds)

I. Triceps Stretch (active flexibility) 5-10 reps (hold for 15 seconds)

J. Triceps Stretch (static flexibility) 10-15 reps

K. Clasping Triceps Stretch 10-15 reps

L. Clasping Rear Delt Stretch 5-10 reps

M. Active Back Flexibility Workout (details later)

Day 2: Back/Biceps (Rest Day)

A. Barbell Deadlift 3 x 8-12 reps

B. Seated Row 3 x 8-12 reps

C. Lat Stretch 5-10 reps (hold for 15 seconds)

D. Bicep Stretch (active flexibility) 5-10 reps (hold for 15 seconds)

E. Bicep Stretch (static flexibility) 10-15 reps

F. Kneeling Overhead Triceps Stretch 10-15 reps

G. Head to Toe Bicep Stretch 10-15 reps

H. Lat Stretch 5-10 reps (hold for 15 seconds)

I. Bicep Stretch (active flexibility) 5-10 reps (hold for 15 seconds)

J. Bicep Stretch (static flexibility) 10-15 reps

K. Kneeling Overhead Triceps Stretch 10-15 reps

L. Head to Toe Bicep Stretch 10-15 reps

M. Lat Stretch 5-10 reps (hold for 15 seconds)

N. Bicep Stretch (active flexibility) 5-10 reps (hold for 15 seconds)

O. Bicep Stretch (static flexibility) 10-15 reps

P. Kneeling Overhead Triceps Stretch 10-15 reps

Q. Head to Toe Bicep Stretch 10-15 reps

Day 3: Legs/Core(Rest Day)

A. Barbell Deadlift 3 x 8-12 reps

B. Leg Press 3 x 8-12 reps

C. Cable Woodchop 2 x 15-20 reps

D. Hip Flexor Stretch 5-10 reps (hold for 15 seconds; each leg)

E. Hamstring Stretch (active flexibility) 5-10 reps (hold for 15 seconds; each leg)

F. Hamstring Stretch (static flexibility) 10-15 reps

G. Quad Stretch 5-10 reps (hold for 15 seconds; each leg)

H. Lat Stretch 5-10 reps (hold for 15 seconds; each leg)

I. Bicep Stretch (active flexibility) 5-10 reps (hold for 15 seconds; each arm)

J. Bicep Stretch (static flexibility) 10-15 reps

K. Kneeling Overhead Triceps Stretch 10-15 reps

L. Clasping Triceps Stretch 10-15 reps

M. Clasping Rear Delt Stretch 5-10 reps

N. Core Flexibility Workout (details later)

Day 4: Chest/Triceps (Rest Day)

A. Flat Barbell Bench Press 3 x 8-12 reps

B. Decline Push Up 2 x 15-20 reps

C. Chest Stretch 5-10 reps (hold for 15 seconds)

D. Tricep Stretch (active flexibility) 5-10 reps (hold for 15 seconds)

E. Tricep Stretch (static flexibility) 10-15 reps

F. Clasping Tricep Stretch 10-15 reps

G. Clasping Rear Delt Stretch 10-15 reps

H. Chest Stretch 5-10 reps (hold for 15 seconds)

I. Tricep Stretch (active flexibility) 5-10 reps (hold for 15 seconds)

J. Tricep Stretch (static flexibility) 10-15 reps

K. Clasping Tricep Stretch 10-15 reps

L. Clasping Rear Delt Stretch 5-10 reps

M. Active Back Flexibility Workout (details later)

Day 5: Back/Biceps (Rest Day)

A. Good Morning 3 x 8-12 reps

B. Deadlift 3 x 8-12 reps

C. Lat Stretch 5-10 reps (hold for 15 seconds; each arm)

D. Bicep Stretch (active flexibility) 5-10 reps (hold for 15 seconds; each arm)

E. Bicep Stretch (static flexibility) 10-15 reps

F. Kneeling Overhead Tricep Stretch 10-15 reps

G. Clasping Front Delt Stretch 10-15 reps

H. Lat Stretch 5-10 reps (hold for 15 seconds; each arm)

I. Bicep Stretch (active flexibility) 5-10 reps (hold for 15 seconds; each arm)

J. Bicep Stretch (static flexibility) 10-15 reps

K. Kneeling Overhead Tricep Stretch 10-15 reps

L. Clasping Front Delt Stretch 5-10 reps

M. Lat Stretch 5-10 reps (hold for 15 seconds; each arm)

N. Bicep Stretch (active flexibility) 5-10 reps (hold for 15 seconds; each arm)

O. Bicep Stretch (static flexibility) 10-15 reps

P. Kneeling Overhead Tricep Stretch 10-15 reps

Q. Clasping Front Delt Stretch 5-10 reps

R. Lat Stretch 5-10 reps (hold for 15 seconds; each arm)

S. Bicep Stretch (active flexibility) 5-10 reps (hold for 15 seconds; each arm)

T. Bicep Stretch (static flexibility) 10-15 reps

U. Kneeling Overhead Tricep Stretch 10-15 reps

V. Clasping Front Delt Stretch 5-10 reps

W. Lat Stretch 5-10 reps (hold for 15 seconds; each arm)

X. Bicep Stretch (active flexibility) 5-10 reps (hold for 15 seconds; each arm)

Y. Bicep Stretch (static flexibility) 10-15 reps

Z. Kneeling Overhead Tricep Stretch 10-15 reps

AA. Clasping Front Delt Stretch 5-10 reps

BB. Lat Stretch 5-10 reps (hold for 15 seconds; each arm)

CC. Bicep Stretch (active flexibility) 5-10 reps (hold for 15 seconds; each arm)

DD. Bicep Stretch (static flexibility) 10-15 reps

EE. Kneeling Overhead Tricep Stretch 10-15 reps

FF. Clasping Front Delt Stretch 5-10 reps

GG. Lat Stretch 5-10 reps (hold for 15 seconds; each arm)

HH. Bicep Stretch (active flexibility) 5-10 reps (hold for 15 seconds; each arm)

II. Bicep Stretch (static flexibility) 10-15 reps

JJ. Kneeling Overhead Tricep Stretch 10-15 reps

KK. Clasping Front Delt Stretch 5-10 reps

LL. Lat Stretch 5-10 reps (hold for 15 seconds; each arm)

MM. Bicep Stretch (active flexibility) 5-10 reps (hold for 15 seconds; each arm)

Chapter 6: Resize Your Thighs

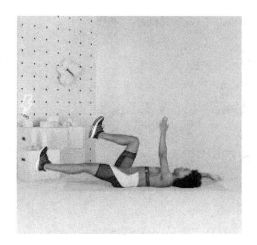

These workouts will focus on your thighs and legs. Although your Full Body Workouts work these muscles, if this is a trouble spot for you in terms of strength, you may want a more targeted routine.

Leg and Thigh Workout 1

This workout is structured as others you have done, organized into Part A and Part B. You will be learning some new exercises, and using some you have already learned.

Part A

Do 10 Squat Jumps are performed safely this way:

Stand with feet together and hands on hips. Keeping your back straight, slowly bend your knees until they are at a 90 degree angle, then thrust upwards, jumping as high as you can. When you land, bring your knees back up to a 90-degree angle. This is one rep.

1. Squats

Stand tall with feet hip-width apart, holding a set of 5- to 15-pound dumbbells at your sides. Slowly bend knees and hips and lower your body until thighs are at least parallel to the floor. Keep head facing forward and chest up. Maintain control of the weights at all times during exercise. Reverse direction to return to starting position and repeat for reps.

2. Lunges

Holding 5- to 15-pound dumbbells in each hand, step forward with left foot and lower body into a lunge until front thigh is parallel to floor; keep back leg straight so that knee does not extend past toe as you go down. Return to start and repeat with right leg. That's 1 rep.

3. Triceps Extensions

Grasp a pair of dumbbells and stand with knees bent and weights hanging at your sides. Straighten arms in front of you until they form a 90-degree angle with your upper arms; keep elbows pointing down toward the floor throughout exercise. Press weights overhead until arms are straight but not locked, then bend elbows to lower them back down. That's 1 rep.

4. Pushups

Start in an elevated pushup position, with hands on the floor directly beneath shoulders, body straight from head to heels, legs extended behind you and toes pointing forward (A). Bend elbows to lower body until chest nearly touches floor (B). Push back up to start and repeat for reps.

5. Squats Alternate with Biceps Curls

Hold a pair of dumbbells in each hand, arms hanging at your sides. Keeping back straight, bend knees and hips as if you were sitting into a chair (A) until thighs are at least parallel to the floor. Now stand and push weights toward ceiling until elbows are fully extended

(B). Reverse movement to return to start and repeat for reps.

Do 10 Side Lunges.

Complete Part A 8 times.

Rest 2 minutes.

Part B
Do 10 Jumping Lunges.

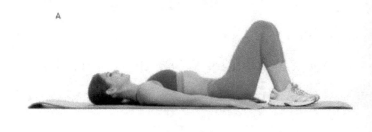

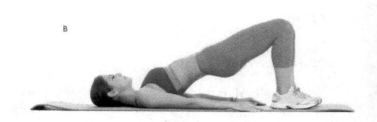

Do 10 Glute Bridges. This is how to do **Glute Bridges:**

1. Lie in neutral position on your back on the floor. A neutral position is not totally flat, nor totally arched. You should be able to slip you hand part way into the curve of your back, but it should not fit all the way.

2. Place your feet, at hip width, evenly on the floor, with your toes pointing forward and your knees bent.

3. Contract your abdominal muscles. Imagine your belly button pulling in toward your spine. Keep your muscles this way throughout the exercise.

4. Push your hips up through your heels. You back should remain in the neutral position. If you back begins to arch or you feel pressure on your neck, you have done too fat.

5. You will keep your abdominals contracted as you lower your hips to the floor.

6. You should not truly rest in between repetitions, only lightly touch the floor.

Complete Part B 8 times.

Rest 2 minutes.

Continue cycling through Parts A and B for 15 minutes.

Leg and Thigh Workout 2

This workout is organized as a circuit. This means that you go from one exercise to another with only a 10 second rest in between. You are measuring by time instead of repetitions, so do each move as quickly and correctly as you can.

Do Squats for 30 seconds

Rest for 10 seconds.

Do Single-Leg Deadlifts for 30 seconds. The **Single-Leg Deadlift** is performed properly this way:

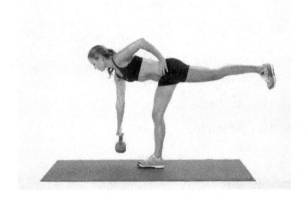

1. Begin in a standing position.

2. Raise one leg straight behind you with your toes pointing downwards.

3. As you raise your leg, bend forward from the hips, keeping your back flat. Keep your neck

aligned with your spine, and loose, not tensed.

4. Your hands will be perpendicular to your chest. Do not reach towards the floor, as this may cause you to round your back.
5. Bend only as far as flexibility will allow, while keeping your core tight and your back straight.
6. Continue with your abs tight and your back straight as you lower your leg and return to a standing position.
7. Do not alternate legs until the next circuit. Stick with the single leg.

Rest 10 seconds.

Do Glute Bridges for 30 seconds.

Rest for 1 minute.

Repeat circuit for the entire 15 minutes. If you can only do a few exercises in the 30 seconds, do not get discouraged. You will get faster.

Lower Body Workout 3

This workout follows the pattern, which should now be familiar to you, of 10 repetitions and Jumping Jacks in between.

Begin with 10 Reverse Lunges.

Then do Jumping Jacks until your timer says 1 minute has passed.

At minute 1, do 10 Side Lunges.

Do Jumping Jacks until minute 2.

At minute 2, Do 10 Squats.

Do Jumping Jacks until minute 3.

At minute 3, do 10 Single-Leg Deadlifts.

Do Jumping Jacks until minute 4.

At minute 4, start again.

Do not forget to switch legs on your Single-Leg Deadlifts when you get there.

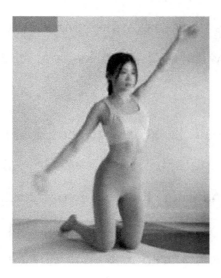

Leg and Thigh Workout 4

This workout will follow the established pattern with Part A and Part B.

Part A

1. Do 10 Jumping Lunges.
2. Rest 10 seconds.
3. Do 10 Single-Leg Deadlifts.
4. Rest 10 seconds.
5. Repeat Part A 8 times.

Part B

1. Do 10 Glute Bridges.
2. Rest 10 seconds.
3. Do 10 Squats.
4. Rest 10 seconds.
5. Repeat Part B 8 times.
6. Cycle between Parts A for the remainder of 15 minutes.

Leg and Thigh Workout 5

This workout is organized as a circuit.

1. Begin with 30 seconds of Jumping Lunges.
2. Rest 10 seconds.
3. Then, do 30 second of Reverse Lunges.
4. Rest 10 seconds.
5. Next, do 30 seconds of Squat Jumps.
6. Rest 1 minute.

Repeat this circuit as many times as you can in 15 minutes.

Chapter 7: The Lean 15-Minute Workouts for Building Muscle and Losing Fat

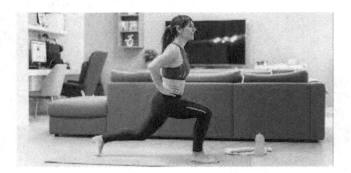

When it comes to building muscle, the biggest obstacle that women face is finding the time to work out. That's why I created The Lean 15 Workouts—the most efficient and effective way for women to burn fat and build lean muscle in only 15 minutes a day. The Lean 15 Workouts take advantage of the body-shaping effects of supersets, which are two exercises performed back-to-back with no rest in between. Supersets force you to work your muscles past their normal failure points, which triggers more growth responses from your body. While you're performing supersets, you'll also be incorporating another muscle-building technique called compound sets, which involve pairing two exercises that work opposing muscle

groups. For example, pairing a bench press with a row works your chest and back.

The Lean 15 Workouts employ both of these strategies in dozens of different combinations to help you build and sculpt your entire body. The best part is that each workout keeps your heart rate elevated throughout the entire routine and you only rest when needed—usually between supersets—so you maximize every second of your workout time. The Lean 15 Workouts are divided into two different types of workouts—The Lean 15 Workouts for Beginners and The Lean 15 Workouts for Experienced Exercisers. Below I explain how to use each workout and provide a sample routine that combines exercises from all four phases of the program.

The Lean 15 Workout for Beginners is designed for women who haven't worked out in a while, are new to weight training, or have never lifted weights before. It's also a good option if you've been exercising regularly with moderate intensity but haven't seen any changes in your body or fitness level. The Lean 15 Workout for Beginners will help you build your strength, endurance, and confidence so you can move on to the next phase of the program. The exercises are broken down into four phases — Phase 1: Resistance Training, Phase 2: Strength Training, Phase 3: Advanced Resistance Training and Phase 4: Strength and Power — and each phase works your body in a slightly different way.

In Phase 1: Resistance Training (weeks 1–4), you'll start out with light weights to get used to the exercises and gradually build up your strength. As your muscles get stronger, you'll gradually increase the amount of weight you lift as well as the number of reps you perform. Phase 1: Resistance Training is a great option if you're just starting out with resistance training or you've been working out regularly but haven't seen any changes in your body. Phase 2: Strength Training (weeks 5–8) focuses on increasing the amount of weight you lift for each exercise. To keep your muscles guessing, we incorporate three different supersets — the kickback superset, the press-up superset and the super squat superset — and alternate between them throughout the routine.

The third phase, Phase 3: Advanced Resistance Training (weeks 9–12), builds on the exercises from Phase 2: Strength Training. We also add another superset — this time the single-arm dumbbell row superset — to keep your body working hard. Phase 4: Strength and Power (weeks 13–16) is a repeat of Phase 2: Strength Training. This time, though, you'll be doing many of the exercises for fewer reps and adding more weight to each exercise.

Phases 1: Resistance Training and 2: Strength Training are great options if you've only been exercising for a few weeks or have never lifted weights before. Both phases will help you build strength, endurance and confidence in the gym so you can graduate to the more advanced exercises in Phase 3: Advanced Resistance Training and Phase 4: Strength and Power. The Lean 15 Workout for Experienced Exercisers is designed for women who have been working out regularly with moderate intensity but haven't seen any changes in their body or fitness level. These workouts focus on increasing your weight-training intensity while maintaining the high-energy, fast-paced workouts that I developed for The Lean 15 Workout for Beginners.

For each of the four phases—Phase 1: Resistance Training, Phase 2: Strength Training, Phase 3: Advanced Resistance Training and Phase 4: Strength and Power—you'll perform one set of each exercise in rapid succession with no rest between exercises. Rest only when needed between supersets (usually after you finish a superset). Each phase is slightly different but all four incorporate supersets into the routine. In Phase 1: Resistance Training (weeks 1–4), for example, you'll alternate between two types of supersets—the press-up superset and the kickback superset—and use dumbbells instead of barbells. In Phase 2: Strength Training (weeks 5–8), you'll perform the same exercises as Phase 1: Resistance Training but this

time we'll use barbells and alternate between three different supersets—the press-up superset, the single-arm dumbbell row superset and the super squat superset.

In Phase 3: Advanced Resistance Training (weeks 9–12) you'll do the same exercises from Phase 2 but with a third superset—the cable pulldown superset. In Phase 4: Strength and Power (weeks 13–16), we'll take it up a notch by performing many of the exercises for fewer reps and adding more weight to each exercise.

Phase 1: Resistance Training is a great option if you've only been exercising for a few weeks or if you haven't lifted weights before. This phase will help you build confidence and get comfortable with the exercises. Phase 2: Strength Training is a great option if you've been working out regularly but haven't seen any changes in your body or fitness level. Phase 2 not only helps you build strength but also focuses on increasing endurance by alternating between different supersets and adding variety to the exercises.

Phase 3: Advanced Resistance Training focuses on increasing your weight-training intensity while maintaining the high-energy, fast-paced workouts that worked so well in Phases 1 and 2. Phase 4: Strength and Power is for experienced exercisers who have been working out regularly with moderate intensity but haven't seen the changes in their body or fitness level that they're looking for. This phase helps you build strength and power so you can graduate to the more advanced exercises in Phase 5: Lean 15 Workout to get the lean, toned body you want.

Phase 1: Resistance Training (weeks 1–4) - Alternate between press-up supersets and kickback supersets, using dumbbells instead of barbells.

Phase 2: Strength Training (weeks 5–8) - Alternate between super squat supersets and single-arm dumbbell row supersets, using barbells instead of dumbbells.

Phase 3: Advanced Resistance Training (weeks 9–12) - Alternate between cable pulldown supersets and super squat supersets, using a variety of weight plates attached to one end of the cable.

Phase 4: Strength and Power (weeks 13–16) - Alternate between walking lunges and squat thrusts.

Phase 5: Lean 15 Workout (weeks 17–20) - Alternate between mountain climbers and glute bridges.

Phase 6: Core Challenge Workout (weeks 21–24) - Alternate between Russian twists and crunches with a medicine ball.

Chapter 8: The 15-Day Body of Your Dreams in Just 15 Minutes a Day (or Less)

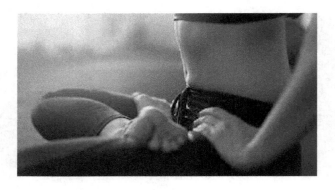

Part I. Introduction to the 15 Day Lean Body Program

The 15 Day Lean Body Program is a variation on the program designed by Martin Rooney and featured in his books. It is ideally suited for those who have a busy schedule but want to stay fit. The 15 Day Lean Body Program uses high intensity interval training (HIIT) to help you build lean muscle mass and burn fat faster than traditional cardio workouts. This quick workout can be done from anywhere with no equipment needed.

The 15 Day Lean Body Program relies on ideal bodyweight exercises to help you build lean muscle mass and burn fat in minimal time. The routines are inspired by the method used by the Australian Army Training Command to train soldiers for fitness and strength, with a specific focus on explosive strength. This method is used by elite athletes around the world.

To get you started, here is a sample routine from the 15 Day Lean Body Program. You can easily follow along with this program in your own home. Feel free to adjust reps or sets, if needed for your fitness level or schedule. Rest as needed between sets and feel free to repeat this workout as many times as you like within a 2-week period. If you need to break up the workout into smaller time periods to accommodate your schedule, that's fine.

• Workout 1 (15 minutes): one set each of squats, lunges, push-ups, and pull-ups

The Bodyweight Cardio Challenge Workout lists the bodyweight cardio exercises that you should use for this 2-week challenge. You will not do burpees because they are a high intensity exercise and therefore you cannot perform them on a day where you will also do bodyweight cardio. Be sure to choose one of the following exercises each time you do bodyweight cardio for the next 14 days.

Workout 2 (15 minutes): Burpee Challenge plus one set of push-ups

The Bodyweight Cardio Challenge Workout lists the bodyweight cardio exercises that you should use for this 2-week challenge. You will not do burpees because they are a high intensity exercise and therefore you cannot perform them on a day where you will also do bodyweight cardio. Be sure to choose one of the following exercises each time you do bodyweight cardio for the next 14 days.

Workout 3 (15 minutes): two sets of each exercise

The Bodyweight Cardio Challenge Workout lists the bodyweight cardio exercises that you should use for this 2-week challenge. You will not do burpees because they are a high intensity exercise and therefore you cannot perform them on a day where you will also do bodyweight cardio. Be sure to choose

one of the following exercises each time you do bodyweight cardio for the next 14 days.

Workout 4 (15 minutes): Bear Challenge plus push-ups

The Bodyweight Cardio Challenge Workout lists the bodyweight cardio exercises that you should use for this 2-week challenge. You will not do burpees because they are a high intensity exercise and therefore you cannot perform them on a day where you will also do bodyweight cardio. Be sure to choose one of the following exercises each time you do bodyweight cardio for the next 14 days.

Workout 5 (15 minutes): Mountain Climber Challenge plus pull-ups

The Bodyweight Cardio Challenge Workout lists the bodyweight cardio exercises that you should use for this 2-week challenge. You will not do burpees because they are a high intensity exercise and therefore you cannot perform them on a day where you will also do bodyweight cardio. Be sure to choose one of the following exercises each time you do bodyweight cardio for the next 14 days.

Part II. The Fast Track to the Core Program

The Fast Track to the Core Program uses high intensity interval training (HIIT) to help you build lean muscle mass and burn fat faster than traditional cardio workouts. This 2-week program can be done from anywhere with no equipment needed.

The Fast Track to the Core Programs relies on ideal bodyweight exercises to help you build lean muscle mass and burn fat in minimal time. The routines are inspired by the method used by the Australian Army Training Command to train soldiers for fitness and strength, with a specific focus on explosive strength. This method is used by elite athletes around the world.

To get you started, here is a sample routine from the Fast Track to the Core Program. You can easily follow along with this program in your own home. Feel free to adjust reps or sets, if needed

for your fitness level or schedule. Rest as needed between sets and feel free to repeat this workout as many times as you like within a 2-week period. If you need to break up the workout into smaller time periods to accommodate your schedule, that's fine.

• Workout 1 (15 minutes): one set each of squats, lunges, push-ups, and pull-ups

The Bodyweight Cardio Challenge Workout lists the bodyweight cardio exercises that you should use for this 2-week challenge. You will not do burpees because they are a high intensity exercise and therefore you cannot perform them on a day where you will also do bodyweight cardio. Be sure to choose one of the following exercises each time you do bodyweight cardio for the next 14 days.

Workout 2 (15 minutes): Burpee Challenge plus one set of push-ups

The Bodyweight Cardio Challenge Workout lists the bodyweight cardio exercises that you should use for this 2-week challenge. You will not do burpees because they are a high intensity exercise and therefore you cannot perform them on a day where you will also do bodyweight cardio. Be sure to choose one of the following exercises each time you do bodyweight cardio for the next 14 days.

Workout 3 (15 minutes): one set of each exercise

The Bodyweight Cardio Challenge Workout lists the bodyweight cardio exercises that you should use for this 2-week challenge. You will not do burpees because they are a high intensity exercise and therefore you cannot perform them on a day where you will also do bodyweight cardio. Be sure to choose one of the following exercises each time you do bodyweight cardio for the next 14 days.

Workout 4 (15 minutes): Bear Challenge plus push-ups

The Bodyweight Cardio Challenge Workout lists the bodyweight cardio exercises that you should use for this 2-week challenge. You will not do burpees

because they are a high intensity exercise and therefore you cannot perform them on a day where you will also do bodyweight cardio. Be sure to choose one of the following exercises each time you do bodyweight cardio for the next 14 days.

Workout 5 (15 minutes): Mountain Climber Challenge plus pull-ups

The Bodyweight Cardio Challenge Workout lists the bodyweight cardio exercises that you should use for this 2-week challenge. You will not do burpees because they are a high intensity exercise and therefore you cannot perform them on a day where you will also do bodyweight cardio. Be sure to choose one of the following exercises each time you do bodyweight cardio for the next 14 days.

Part III. The Fast Track to the Fat Burn Program

The Fast Track to the Fat Burn Program uses high intensity interval training (HIIT) to help you build lean muscle mass and burn fat faster than traditional cardio workouts. This 2-week program can be done from anywhere with no equipment needed."

The Fast Track to the Fat Burn Program relies on ideal bodyweight exercises to help you build lean muscle mass and burn fat in minimal time. The routines are inspired by the method used by the Australian Army Training Command to train soldiers for fitness and strength, with a specific focus on explosive strength. This method is used by elite athletes around the world.

To get you started, here is a sample routine from the Fast Track to the Fat Burn Program. You can easily follow along with this program in your own home. Feel free to adjust reps or sets, if needed for your fitness level or schedule. Rest as needed between sets and feel free to repeat this workout as many times as you like within a 2-week period. If you need to break up the workout into smaller time periods to accommodate your schedule, that's fine.

• Workout 1 (15 minutes): one set each of squats, lunges, push-ups, and pull-ups

The Bodyweight Cardio Challenge Workout lists the bodyweight cardio exercises that you should use for this 2-week challenge. You will not do burpees because they are a high intensity exercise and therefore you cannot perform them on a day where you will also do bodyweight cardio. Be sure to choose one of the following exercises each time you do bodyweight cardio for the next 14 days.

Workout 2 (15 minutes): Burpee Challenge plus one set of push-ups

The Bodyweight Cardio Challenge Workout lists the bodyweight cardio exercises that you should use for this 2-week challenge. You will not do burpees because they are a high intensity exercise and therefore you cannot perform them on a day where you will also do bodyweight cardio. Be sure to choose one of the following exercises each time you do bodyweight cardio for the next 14 days.

Workout 3 (15 minutes): one set of each exercise

The Bodyweight Cardio Challenge Workout lists the bodyweight cardio exercises that you should use for this 2-week challenge. You will not do burpees because they are a high intensity exercise and therefore you cannot perform them on a day where you will also do bodyweight cardio. Be sure to choose one of the following exercises each time you do bodyweight cardio for the next 14 days.

Part IV. Wrapping Up with Fat-Burning Tips from Our All-Star Team

The Fat Burning Plan contains four fat burning workouts to help you create lean muscle mass and burn fat in minimal time. The routines in the program are inspired by the method used by the Australian Army Training Command to train soldiers for fitness and strength, with a specific focus on explosive strength. This method is used by elite athletes around the world.

To get you started, here is a sample routine from the Fat Burning Plan. You can easily follow along with this program in your own home. Feel free to

adjust reps or sets, if needed for your fitness level or schedule. Rest as needed between sets and feel free to repeat this workout as many times as you like within a 2-week period. If you need to break up the workout into smaller time periods to accommodate your schedule, that's fine.

• Workout 1 (15 minutes): one set each of squats, lunges, push-ups, and pull-ups

The Bodyweight Cardio Challenge Workout lists the bodyweight cardio exercises that you should use for this 2-week challenge. You will not do burpees because they are a high intensity exercise and therefore you cannot perform them on a day where you will also do bodyweight cardio. Be sure to choose one of the following exercises each time you do bodyweight cardio for the next 14 days.

Workout 2 (15 minutes): Burpee Challenge plus one set of push-ups

The Bodyweight Cardio Challenge Workout lists the bodyweight cardio exercises that you should use for this 2-

week challenge. You will not do burpees because they are a high intensity exercise and therefore you cannot perform them on a day where you will also do bodyweight cardio. Be sure to choose one of the following exercises each time you do bodyweight cardio for the next 14 days.

Workout 3 (15 minutes): Bear Challenge plus push-ups

The Bodyweight Cardio Challenge Workout lists the bodyweight cardio exercises that you should use for this 2-week challenge. You will not do burpees because they are a high intensity exercise and therefore you cannot perform them on a day where you will also do bodyweight cardio. Be sure to choose one of the following exercises each time you do bodyweight cardio for the next 14 days.

Workout 4 (15 minutes): Mountain Climber Challenge plus pull-ups

The Bodyweight Cardio Challenge Workout lists the bodyweight cardio exercises that you should use for this 2-

week challenge. You will not do burpees because they are a high intensity exercise and therefore you cannot perform them on a day where you will also do bodyweight cardio. Be sure to choose one of the following exercises each time you do bodyweight cardio for the next 14 days.

Chapter 9: Benefits Of 15 Minutes Workout

- One cannot complain that one does not have time to work out, in the busy schedule of life. 15 minutes robust workout technique is commonly being practiced by the working professionals to maintain their work life balance.

- The interval workout with high intensity is said to show better results as compared to normal cardio workout outs which stretch for longer duration.

- The person can decide the kind of work out one wants to plan, to suit his daily needs and his body characteristics.

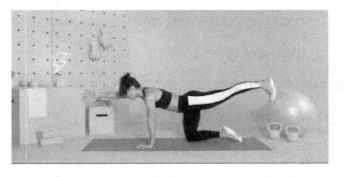

There Are Various Tips Which Needs To Be Followed Before Exercising

1. Start Slow

Any new thing has to be started with lower expectations as it takes time to get used to doing something new and also takes time to get results out of the same. For a start, one should do very basic exercises like running for 10 minutes on a daily basis for next three weeks. Body will need to get used to physical pressure and exercise. If someone starts with a heavy work out then he can seriously damage his internal organs because of excessive heat and sudden increase in body temperature.

2. Change The Cycle

The exercise should be a onetime permanent set. The exercise should keep changing so that it does not get boring and monotonous. According to the purpose of the exercise one should also change the type and duration of exercise. For example if someone wants to increase the body muscle then he should limit his cardio exercise to a bare minimum and if someone is working out to get lean then his whole workout session should be dedicated to cardio exercises. In cardio exercises also one should take care of alternating the exercise on a daily basis. The person exercising in home can change the options from cycling to rowing to running on a treadmill, for 15 minutes.

3.   Separate Cardio From Strength Training

There are various strength building exercises and many cardio exercises which affects separately to the body. The cardio exercises affect the fat of the body and the strength gaining exercises are specific to body parts. If the person wants to gain strength in his hand or legs then he accordingly does crunches and squats to increasing the leg strength. Now running and cycling also is leg exercise but comes under cardio exercise.

It is important to separate the two exercises and do not perform cardio exercise and leg strength increasing exercise in one day. This will lead to fatigue and the purpose of the exercise will not be solved.

4.   Removal Of Fat Burning Zone Myth

Initially it was a common believe that a person need to exercise in 70-80 percent of his maximum heart rate to start the metabolism process and start losing fat. It was also a common believe that one will have to keep working out, in the above mentioned rate, for at least 20 minutes before the fat burning process starts. This, however, has been proven as a myth and now it is accepted that if a person follows interval workout sessions then he can definitely reduce his fat. The interval workout says that the workout should be done on various sessions of 15 minutes. This 15 minute session should be very intense and then after the session a person should take some rest. The metabolism process starts in those 15 minutes.

5.   Practice Low Impact Exercise

There are a few exercises like running on asphalt floor or skipping. These exercises leave a lot of impact on the muscles of the body specially the feet muscles. These exercises lead to muscle breakage and it tears down the stamina to work out more. It is advisable to do intensive exercise but a low impact one. The exercises of this nature are cycling, swimming and running on elliptical machines.

6.   15 Minutes Interval Workouts

To reduce fat early one should to cling to interval workouts. These are the short and heavy sessions of workouts. In a shorter span of time one can lose more as compared to the regular cardio workouts. If a person does 20-30 minutes of interval workout, 2-3 times in a week then he reduces more as compares to 30-60 minutes of daily cardio workouts. The best part of interval workouts is that one keeps losing the body fat even after the workout session is not in the progress. The fat metabolism process is alleviated and it keeps happening for 48 hours after the work out session.

7.   Change The Pattern And Time

Our body gets used to a workout. If a person is doing a particular kind of exercise at one particular time, on each and every single day, then the exercise will stop showing results after sometime. Let us take an example to understand it better. If a person is doing 3 sets of 10 squats each at 8am in morning, on a daily basis then after a month or so the body will get used to the pressure of 10 squats at 8am and thus will stop showing any results. That is why it is advised that a person should keep changing the number of sets he is doing, change the time of exercise and also the kind of exercise, from time to time. The change will give better results.

8.   Body Toning In Interval Exercise

After the 15 minutes exercise session, all the stubborn fat is reduces and the skin is not visible as a loose skin. The interval workouts help in development of muscle in place of fats. This is the reason that, even after burning lot of fat the skin becomes tight as it has been transformed into muscles.

9. Exercise In Cool Area

It is commonly known and accepted that a person cannot exercise a lot in high degree temperature an. It is advised that the exercise should be done in cooler areas. If at all a person has to work out in high degree then he can cool his temperature around his neck and can work out for more time even in high degree. Wear an ice strap around neck region or wear a wet handkerchief around a neck region and run in treadmill. The duration will definitely increase vis s vis non cooling exercise.

10. Wear Comfortable Clothes

During work out wear something which does not absorb heat from outside and store in the body. for example if someone wear black color clothes during workout then this color cloth will absorb all the radiation from sun and will not reflect back. This will increase the heat within the body. The body is anyways heated up because of heavy workout and then if it socks more heat from outside then it will be dangerous for body. One should always take care of clothes and wear loose and light color clothes.

Conclusion

You now have the tools to workout without worrying about travelling or having access to a gym. You can workout anywhere at anytime. All you need is your bodyweight and determination. With these workouts, you can take your fitness to the next level by learning how to get fit, lean muscle mass and burn fat faster than traditional cardio workouts with minimal time.

You will be amazed at what your body is capable of doing when you challenge yourself with new workouts for fat burning. These workouts will help you burn maximum calories and get lean muscle mass too! If you would like to learn more about the secrets of fat burning then go here my website Bodyweight Cardio Training. You will learn more about fat burning workouts without needing to spend hours on the treadmill or run on a track. You can get fit without having to spend hours a day. You will learn the secrets of bodyweight cardio training to get lean muscle mass and burn fat in minimal time. So why wait. It's time to start your bodyweight cardio challenge now. Goodbye boring workouts for fat burning! Hello bodyweight cardio training for lean muscle mass and fat burning.

HYPNOSIS FOR WEIGHT LOSS

By

Lil Ron

Table of Contents

Introduction

Hypnosis, a practice often referred to as hypnotherapy, refers to a form of guided relaxation that combines a state of intense focus with heightened concentration. It is a practice that has been described as placing the mind in a trance state. While one may jump to the conclusion that it has the same relaxation effects on the brain like a drug, such as cannabis, there's an instance of induced concentration that affects the mind oppositely compared to any other mind-altering drug.

During hypnosis or hypnotherapy, which is only recommended to be carried out by a professional physician, the mind is blocked from the world. In the state of hypnosis, one cannot register their surroundings as they are placed in an incredibly deep state of concentration. This state of mind shouldn't be broken unless it is done so intentionally by a hypnotherapist.

Traditionally, when placed under hypnotherapy, the individual's attention is centered and based on preference and can be placed in different instances, which mainly involves activating selective memories. However, even though this was the initial use of the practice, it has evolved into a now, broadly-marketed relaxation experience that can benefit the physical body, cognitive function, and increase mental well-being.

Modern-day hypnosis has been around since the late 18th Century and was popularized by a German physician dubbed the father of hypnotism, Franz Mesmer.

Although the practice has been around for over a century and society has been aware of it for a long time, not many people understand what it entails. Some even draw their own conclusions.

Reading the title, "Hypnosis for weight loss," you probably didn't know someone could lose weight engaging in hypnotherapy. Although it's not a topic that has been idealized or highlighted as a solution to weight loss, it has proven to be effective. Taking a look at most conditions and ailments, you'll come to find that the majority is related to stress, including the increased risk of infection, a state of bodily imbalance, or simply being faced with symptoms throughout your daily life that you perceive as common and normal.

Symptoms like rapid weight gain or perhaps not being able to lose weight at all, to poor digestion and water retention, there are more contributing factors than meets the eye in correlation with possibly just living an unhealthy lifestyle. These symptoms are extremely common. It contributes to many adverse health issues and, of course, has become normalized symptoms in our everyday lives.

Referring to the term "normalized symptoms," we're referring to an occurrence of symptoms displayed by your body that may make you feel uncomfortable, fatigued and overall, unwell.

Regardless of what society may think they know or don't know about the practice at all, hypnosis can invite many benefits into your life, such as:

- Relieve your mind of anxiety, depression, and fear
- Reduce or eliminate the symptoms associated with stress
- Tap into and heal sleep disorders
- Manage post-trauma anxiety and help you cope with loss
- Treat stress or conditions related to stress, such as smoking and substance abuse
- Help you lose weight effectively and permanently

Chapter 1:

Hypnosis and Hypnotherapy

Hypnosis and hypnotherapy are often described as being one in the same practice, but they are not.

Hypnotherapy is a type of guided hypnosis that mainly focuses on concentration, while hypnosis refers to the act of guiding an individual into a trance state of mind. With hypnosis, this state is commonly referred to as either a resting state of relaxation, induced suggestibility, or hyperfocus.

Something the average student or working individual battles with every day is to keep focus during their daily routine. A consistent lack of focus may leave an individual feeling tired, unmotivated, stressed, and inefficient. That's just one of the main reasons why hypnotherapy serves as the ultimate solution for anyone looking to improve productivity, relieve stress and anxiety, and boost their overall health.

Hypnotherapy is used in various instances, all of which have been proven to be very effective. It is similar to other types of psychological treatments with benefits that are similar to that of psychotherapy.

The practice treats conditions, including phobias, anxiety disorders, bad habits, weight gain, substance abuse, learning disorders, poor communication skills, and can even treat pain. It can resolve digestive and gastrointestinal disorders, as well as severe hormonal skin disorders, aiding as a massive solution to many different issues people face daily and are often unaware of how to treat.

Many patients with immune disorders or severe conditions, such as cancer, can also be treated with hypnotherapy as it is known for its pain-relieving abilities. It is especially helpful and used when patients undergo chemotherapy or physical rehabilitation that is excessively painful.

Hypnotherapy is carried out by a therapist in a therapeutic and tranquil environment that allows the patient to enter and remain in a focused state of mind. Apart from its incredible benefits, it can adjust the mind and shift mental behavior, almost tricking the brain into focusing on positive intentions. Often, with severe cases, such as advanced stages of cancer, patients are almost convinced that they are not going to live very long. Some may even receive their expected date of passing from their medical practitioner.

Faced with extreme negativity, such as a patient being told that they are going to die, patients tend to give up.

Now, regardless of what you believe, what your mind conceives to believe may very well become a reality. This manner of thinking holds a lot of truth and could set a patient apart from surviving their condition. Although it is difficult to achieve a state of mind where one is positive when faced with illness, hypnotherapy can indeed adjust one's thought process and retrain the brain into thinking only positive thoughts.

In essence, a cancer patient's attitude can massively contribute to their probability of healing. Hypnotherapy can, in fact, relieve not only pain but also add a mental shield against negative thinking processes that could contribute to a patient's inability to recover.

From various types of recovery, acting as more than just a supportive release for pain, emotional and mental stability, something many individuals find fascinating is that one can lose weight with hypnotherapy.

Depending on the severity of the problem being treated, hypnotherapy may take longer to see a difference. Upon meeting with a hypnotherapist, the practitioner will assess the extent of hypnotherapy required, measured in hours, for the patient to obtain the result they would like to see at the end of their course of therapy. A specific total number of hours will be prescribed to the patient, forming a part of alternative healthcare.

Take it as a tip, with hypnotherapy it is very important to feel comfortable with your practitioner, which is why you must seek out several just to find the right one. With hypnotherapy, it's always a good idea to ask around for recommendations and not settle for the first therapist you come across.

Since you now have a good understanding of hypnotherapy, it's necessary also to be informed about hypnosis.

Hypnosis, as previously mentioned, refers to placing an individual in a trance state of mind, also referred to as deep relaxation, increased suggestibility and hyperfocus.

Thinking about the different references related to hypnosis, one may think of it as being a focused-based of deep sleep. When we sleep, we tend to enter and exit a trance state quite often. This can also occur when we listen to music or when we are focused on reading a book or watching a movie. It invites a state of mind where our thought processes almost come to a halt as we are focused, and our brain suddenly even more so than it is used to. Whenever you immerse yourself into something and focus, you enter a trance state of mind.

So, what's the difference between professional hypnosis, the actual act of induced hypnosis, and our brief everyday moments of intense focus?

Well, about the only difference is that with hypnosis, you are assisted with a hypnotherapist to enter a trance state of mind where you can achieve wonderful things. You can achieve a state of motivation, positivity, healing, stress-relief, and even weight loss.

The Myths:

Those who believe in myths or are superstitious have painted a picture of hypnosis that has managed to scare people away.

Whether you've heard about hypnosis in the media, saw it in a movie or were shunned by your parents against learning more about it, you can rest assured that it's not as bad as society makes it out to be.

Can hypnotists control the minds of their patients? Of course not. Hypnosis is used as a medical practice to either relieve symptoms associated with pain, anxiety, or help people to lose weight and get back on the healthy train again. It doesn't leave you feeling helpless or unaware of what you're doing.

During hypnotherapy, patients are still conscious and can hear everything that is happening around them, which is another reason why it is considered an entirely safe practice. To assure people

even more, it is next to impossible for anyone to be unconscious when undergoing hypnosis.

Differentiating between hypnosis and hypnotherapy, you now have learned that both practices have a similar foundation yet can help patients achieve different goals. Both practices can indeed help patients lose weight.

When you want to lose weight, you have to focus on different things. Losing weight is never just about cleaning up your diet and incorporating exercise into your daily routine.

Since stress is a major part of the reason why our bodies hold onto weight, hypnosis serves as the perfect solution to relieve stress and can also manage disorders often contributing to weight gain. This includes both anxiety and depression. Additionally, it can help individuals with either an overactive or underactive thyroid to reach some level of balance, allowing one's body to lose weight permanently and sustainably.

Hypnotherapy, on the other hand, is perfect for treating many different cases, including bad habits like smoking and overeating, which can contribute to a variety of eating disorders. Both can help you develop a bad relationship with food and even act as a means of coping with stress. That is why hypnosis and hypnotherapy can work hand-in-hand to achieve attainable results, depending on your needs. Hypnotherapy also relieves mind-body illnesses and reduces symptoms, including irritable bowel syndrome, skin conditions, and various types of addictions.

Unless you suffer from severe stress-related disorders that require you to engage in both practices, hypnotherapy can serve all of your needs concerning weight loss. It is the perfect option for anyone aiming to achieve long-term results.

Given that every decision, thought and intention is birthed in the mind, it's quite simple to see why hypnotherapy can solve a lot of the problems we as humans face with our bodies today.

Hypnosis for weight loss has been suggested as being both effective and not at all effective. According to studies conducted in the 90s, patients lost twice the amount of weight than on a given diet (Lefave, June 28,2019).

Another study, conducted in 2014, included 60 women suffering from obesity. The study proved that hypnotherapy can aid in every individual's weight loss and even improved their body image and eating habits. After the successful completion of their diets combined with hypnotherapy, none were required to reduce fat surgically (Psychology Today, Dec. 20, 2014).

Both hypnosis and hypnotherapy serve as practices that help deplete negative habits and can assist anyone, no matter how sick or unmotivated, to get back on track, follow a healthy diet and attainable exercise program, as well as kick many harmful addictions.

Hypnosis for Weight Loss: The Golden Method of Burning Fat Quickly and Permanently Through Hypnosis

Since we've already debunked the conspiracy theories on whether hypnosis is a form of mind-control practiced by individuals with hidden agendas, let's dive right into all of the hype that surrounds the idea of its effectivity.

Hypnosis plays an important role in medicinal solutions. In modern-day society, it is recommended for treating many different conditions, including obesity or weight loss in individuals who are overweight. It also serves patients who have undergone surgery extremely well, particularly if they are restricted from exercising after surgery. Given that it is the perfect option for losing weight, it is additionally helpful to anyone who is disabled or recovering from an injury.

Once you understand the practice and how it is conducted, you will find that everything makes sense. Hypnosis works for weight loss because of the relationship between our minds and bodies. Without proper communication being relayed from our minds to our bodies, we would not be able to function properly. Since hypnosis allows the brain to adopt new ideas and habits, it can help push anyone in the right direction and could potentially improve our quality of living.

Adopting new habits can help eliminate fear, improve confidence, and inspire you to maintain persistence and a sense of motivation on your weight loss journey. Since two of the biggest issues society faces today are media-based influences and a lack of motivation, you can easily solve any related issues by simply correcting your mind.

Correcting your mind is an entirely different mission on its own, or without hypnosis, that is. It is a challenge that most get frustrated with. Nobody wants to deal with themselves. Although that may be true, perhaps one of the best lessons hypnosis teaches you is the significance of spending time focusing on your intentions. Practicing hypnosis daily includes focusing on certain ideas. Once these ideas are normalized in your daily routine and life, you will find it easier to cope with struggles and ultimately break bad habits, which is the ultimate goal.

In reality, it takes 21 consecutive days to break a bad habit but only if a person remains persistent, integrating both a conscious and consistent effort to quit or rectify a habit. It takes the same amount of time to adopt a new healthy habit. With hypnosis, it can take up to three months to either break a bad habit or form a new one. However, even though hypnosis takes longer, it tends to work far more effectively than just forcing yourself to do something you don't want to do.

Our brains are powerful operating systems that can be fooled under the right circumstances. Hypnosis has been proven to be effective for breaking habits and adopting new ones due to its powerful effect on the mind. It can be measured in the same line of consistency and power as affirmations. Now, many would argue that hypnosis is unnecessary and that completing a 90-day practice of hypnotherapy to change habits for weight loss is a complete waste of time. However, when you think about someone who needs to lose weight but can't seem to do it, then you might start reconsidering it as a helpful solution to the problem. It's no secret that the human brain requires far more than a little push or single affirmation to thrive. Looking at motivational video clips and reading quotes daily is great, but is it really helping you to move further than from A to B?

It's true that today, we are faced with a sense of rushing through life. Asking an obese or unhealthy individual why they gained weight, there's a certainty that you'll receive similar answers.

Could it be that no one has time to, for instance, cook or prep healthy meals, visit the gym or simply move their bodies? Apart from making up excuses as to why you can't do something, there's actual evidence hidden in the reasons why we sell ourselves short and opt for the easy way out.

Could it be that the majority of individuals have just become lazy?

Regardless of your excuses, reasons or inabilities, hypnosis debunks the idea that you have to go all out to get healthier. Losing weight to improve your physical appearance has always been a challenge, and although there is no easy way out, daily persistence and 10 to 60 minutes a day of practice could help you to lose weight. Not just that, but it can also restructure your brain and help you to develop better habits, which will guide you in experiencing a much more positive and sustainable means of living.

Regardless of the practice or routine you follow at the end of the day, the principle of losing weight always remains the same. You have to follow a balanced diet in proportion with a sustainable exercise routine.

By not doing so is where most people tend to go wrong with their weight loss journeys. It doesn't matter whether it's a diet supplement, weight loss tea, or even hypnosis. Your diet and exercise routine still plays an increasingly important role in losing weight and will be the number one factor that will help you to obtain permanent results. There's a lot of truth in the advice given that there aren't any quick fixes to help you lose weight faster than what's recommended. Usually, anything that promotes standard weight loss, which is generally about two to five pounds a week, depending on your current Body Mass Index (BMI), works no matter what it is. The trick to losing weight doesn't necessarily lie in what you do, but rather in how you do it.

When people start with hypnosis, they may be very likely to quit after a few days or weeks, as it may not seem useful or it isn't leading to any noticeable results.

Nevertheless, if you remain consistent with it, eat a balanced diet instead of crash dieting, and follow a simple exercise routine, then you will find that it has a lot more to offer you than just weight loss. Even though weight loss is the goal of this book, it's important to keep in mind that lasting results don't occur overnight. There are no quick fixes, especially with hypnosis.

Adopting the practice, you will discover many benefits, yet two of the most important ones are healing and learning how to activate the fat burning process inside of your body.

Healing the body with hypnosis

Hypnosis is a practice used for losing weight, but since healing forms an essential part of retraining both the body and mind to perform in perfect harmony, it needs to be treated as a tool to calm the mind. Once you've mastered the art of self-control, you can move on and easily convince yourself that you are capable of losing weight, reaching your goal weight, and achieving many other fitness goals that you once thought wasn't possible.

Losing weight is a time-consuming process. The more weight you have to lose, the more patience and persistence you need to become successful. In that same breath, if you've got a lot of weight to lose, it's most likely that you will also have to address certain health issues. Integrating hypnosis into your daily routine can reduce stress and help obtain a sense of regularity and balance, which is required to lose weight. Medically speaking, since hypnosis treats stress too, it is perfect for anyone suffering from obesity, eating disorders, an overactive or underactive thyroid, or anyone who struggles to follow a healthy, balanced diet.

Fat burning activation with hypnosis

Hypnosis is not a diet, nor is it a fast-track method to get you where you want to go. Instead, it is a tool used to help individuals reach their goals by implementing proper habits. These habits can help you achieve results by focusing on proper diet and exercise. Since most weight-related issues are influenced by psychological issues, hypnosis acts as the perfect tool, laying a foundation for a healthy mind.

Hypnosis is not a type of mind control, yet it is designed to alter your mind by shifting your feelings toward liking something that you might have hated before, such as exercise or eating a balanced diet. The same goes for quitting sugar or binge eating. Hypnosis identifies the root of the issues you may be dealing with and works by rectifying it accordingly. Given that it changes your thought pattern, you may also experience a much calmer and relaxed approach to everything you do.

Hypnosis works by maintaining changes made in the mind because of neuroplasticity. Consistent hypnotherapy sessions create new patterns in the brain that result in the creation of new habits. Since consistency is the number one key to losing weight, it acts as a solution to overcome barriers in your mind, which is something the majority of individuals struggle with.

Hypnosis can also provide you with many techniques to meet different goals, such as gastric band hypnosis, which works by limiting eating habits, causing you to refrain from overeating.

Is hypnosis the answer to reach your weight loss goals?

Hypnosis is not a medical procedure, so it doesn't require a medical practitioner to be carried out successfully. In fact, you can even do it yourself at home. However, if you're looking for proper results or would like to achieve substantial goals, including quitting an addiction, reducing pain or treat obesity, it may be better to seek help from a professional.

If you're just doing it to shed extra pounds, you can easily do it by yourself. Hypnosis works for anyone looking for a solution to kick their bad habits and adopt new ones. It can act as a method that can get you to where you want to go faster and can benefit every individual as we all seem to struggle with something in our everyday lives.

Evidence that hypnosis is useful

The best way to describe the experience of hypnosis is to view it as a type of therapy that focuses on controlled attention. It's not something that feels scary or out of the ordinary. Those who are apprehensive should consider giving it a shot at least once before debunking the practice altogether. It's something that can benefit you by allowing you to change your habits healthily.

Is there a negative side to hypnosis? It depends on how you perceive the practice, as well as additional features it encompasses.

For some, it may be a wonderful experience, but for others, not. Since it's not an invasive procedure, and you're not taking something physically to lose weight, it may come across as a fad. If you're the type of person who struggles to stick to something or can't see beyond what's in front of you, then chances are it may not be your cup of tea.

Also, unless you have the willpower to engage in self-hypnosis consistently, you will have to visit a hypnotherapist to receive hypnotherapy sessions. Professional sessions can cost anywhere between $100 to $250 an hour. Considering that you have to engage in hypnosis for at least three months to see proper results, it's easy to see why people may quit at the get-go. Since most insurance companies refrain from covering hypnosis, it will also have to come out of your pocket.

On a positive note, if you can't afford professional hypnotherapy sessions, you can find countless guides, articles, and podcasts like this one online. If you can manage to put in the necessary time required to succeed in losing weight or simply kick some of your bad habits, then you will be thrilled to find that it is indeed very effective. Although three months of practice seems incredibly long, you will reach your goals in no time. Plus, you'll do it in a sustainable self-sufficient manner, which is also a bonus for your self-development.

Often, when people can't lose weight, it is because they are unmotivated and deprived of a positive and disciplined mindset.

Hypnosis manages to target specific factors that cause weight gain. In a sustainable manner, hypnosis helps you overcome those negative influencing factors, which can present itself as quite challenging to face daily.

Challenges may include anxiety disorders, depression, stress, fear, negative eating habits, such as overeating or consuming a low-calorie diet and addictive habits, such as smoking and consuming alcohol.

Hypnosis is a passive-aggressive approach to solving problems people face in their daily lives, but generally they don't know how to deal with them. It alters our minds to change the way we respond and react, and can aid as a healthy tool to guide us through our daily struggles, worries, and just about any situation with ease. Since unmindful

eating, such as overeating or even a bulimic disorder, are usually influenced by emotional reactions, it's becoming clear why hypnosis could work for those who suffer from any type of related disorder. Adding self-image into the mix, it's equally understandable why a person's self-image can be rectified with hypnotherapy. Once the individual's mind is altered to accept themselves, care for themselves and treat their bodies as something valuable, only then will they be inclined to take better care of themselves. This goes hand-in-hand with what they consume every day and the effort they are more likely to put in to feel good and not only look good.

Focusing on the right things, such as health rather than image, can shift your mindset significantly. It's like focusing on making money in your career instead of obtaining overall happiness in your life. If you're not happy, then making money will just be a temporary escape or solution to your problems. However, if you spend time doing what you love and are really passionate about it, instead of doing something you potentially don't like because you're making money from it, the long-term results will be quite negative. Since we only get one body, one machine to operate with, we as humans must be inclined to look after it.

People are also more likely to find it difficult to maintain a healthy lifestyle if they have low self-esteem.

This contributes to the reason why hypnosis is so effective, and considering that you can do it all by yourself instead of seeing a hypnotherapist, gives you no excuse to not engage in some manner of self-healing through hypnotherapy. It can be just as effective carried out by yourself as it is presented by a professional.

By adopting a healthier mind to consume better food and improve your lifestyle, also comes the responsibility to learn more about healthy living. Even if you're in the healthy mindset of wanting to eat a balanced diet, what do you actually know about doing it? Sure, every day we are presented with countless advertising campaigns and food products that pushes the following terms:

- Low fat
- No sugar
- 25+ added vitamins
- Low caloric deficit

However, are these disclaimers really what we should be looking for on the packaging labels of our food?

Not whatsoever. The last thing you should be eating is artificially-induced foods, with package labels that suggest that vitamins or minerals has been added to it. The same goes for the label "no sugar." We don't know whether you've given it a thought, but why does that yogurt taste so sweet?

Is it magic? Well, of course not, but it has definitely been pumped with something that's not good for you. Some of the most common artificial sweeteners include aspartame and xylitol, which can have serious negative effects on your long-term health if consumed daily. Yet food brands don't disclaim that on their labels, do they?

When undergoing hypnotherapy with the purpose of becoming healthier or to lose weight, you can't just visit your hypnotherapist or conduct the session yourself. You have to implement a process that will support new intentions, such as eating healthier. There are countless eBooks, podcasts, and cookbooks available online and in-store to help you to maintain a sustainable diet. If you're really uncertain about what to do, it's always a good idea to ask your medical practitioner. Having your blood tested for certain allergies or intolerances, such as dairy, glucose, and wheat can also be quite helpful in guiding you with what you should and shouldn't eat.

The best way to lose weight, of course, is to maintain a consistent balance of 80% nutrition and 20% physical activity. To lose weight effectively and permanently with hypnosis, you have to follow the 80:20 rule ratio.

Hypnosis works for weight loss, but only if you devote yourself and maintain a healthy balanced lifestyle. Again, it's important to remember that hypnosis is not a diet or quick solution that will get you to where you want to be. Instead, it's a tool that can be used to support your weight loss journey by rectifying old habits and possibly creating new sustainable ones.

Providing you with raw evidence of someone losing weight as a result of hypnosis by displaying a before and after photo isn't a very reasonable tactic, either.

Anyone can post pictures online and promote a weight loss method. However, trying it out, you'll start to notice a more mindful version of yourself, which won't only translate in your relationship on how to approach food, exercise or your lifestyle, but it will also show in the way you treat and take care of yourself.

At the end of the day, our bodies serve as vessels that carry us through life. How well we look after it, is entirely up to us.

Chapter 2:

Hypnosis Weight Loss Session

Welcome to the weight loss hypnosis session, which can be conducted in the comfort of your home or just about anywhere you won't be likely to experience interruptions. Given that hypnosis requires you to be completely focused on your thoughts, preferably in silence, you will need to find a space where this is attainable.

Getting rid of potentially interrupting objects, such as your smartphone or any digital device and noise is necessary for you to take in the complete experience. Without focus, you will not be able to access a quiet space in your mind and will be constantly distracted.

Apart from physical surroundings and creating a tranquil or quiet environment, it's also best to ensure you practice hypnosis for weight loss without people around or any noise. It's also best to choose a space where you feel safe and content before you start your practice. Returning to this space every day around the same time will help you to develop the habit of practicing hypnosis daily and stick to a routine. Without consistency, hypnosis won't produce the necessary results required to aid in your weight loss journey. All these factors are important to take note of before starting your hypnosis for weight-loss session.

Since you're reading this, you are obviously interested in what hypnosis for weight loss has to offer you, and given that you've chosen weight loss as a specified solution to help you in your daily life, good for you to decide to implement change.

Although kickstarting a journey like this, whether it's 21-days or up to three months, may seem difficult to follow through until the end, I hope this session will inspire you to keep coming back for more.

This session includes a 21-day guided meditation plan, which is specifically designed to help you develop a habit. After these three weeks, you are more likely to want to engage in some form of hypnotherapy daily as it will have proven to serve you positively.

That's the thing with doing something really beneficial for you, much like hypnosis, often, you are hesitant to do it unless you've managed to develop a routine. This routine must, of course, be sustainable and in some sense either enjoyable or feel like it's positively affecting your day. The same goes for exercising, your daily eating habits, and any methods you may implement to rid your body and mind of stress.

Now, although 21-days of benefiting your physical health and mental well-being doesn't necessarily present itself as a challenge, most individuals can't commit to any practice that lasts as long as three weeks. However, if you take a moment to consider the benefits you will reap after three weeks, even entering the habitual period thereafter, it may become easier to adopt hypnosis as a part of your daily routine toward healthy living.

Given that hypnosis is focused on creating new habits and replacing bad ones, you'll find that it can be quite addictive once you've managed to quiet your mind. We, as humans, most definitely require some time to wind down and destress after busy days spent in the midst of stress, which persists all throughout our lives. In today's fast-paced world, it's very uncommon to not experience some form of stress, anxiety, or even depression in our lives. Stress specifically, is one of the biggest contributing factors why people gain weight.

Hypnosis is often compared to meditating. Looking at the similarities, it's easy to see why this makes sense. Since people often struggle to meditate, with the main issue being struggling to calm their minds, hypnosis may present itself as a difficult challenge to start.

However, with persistence, this will surely get better. Something is changing your attitude and the way you perceive different factors in your life, including the difficulty of quieting your mind,

which can spark significant change in your reality.

This, of course, is not "The Secret," yet it has countless similarities and characteristics that present the same outcome for those who try it. If you think about what causes you to develop bad habits, you will find that it is primarily stress or teachings instilled in you from a young age. If you think about what causes you to overeat, as an example, you would easily believe that hypnosis can indeed lead you to turn that habit around.

Since we tend to rush through our daily lives, including work and our duties at home, we don't slow down to take the time to look after ourselves.

There are a lot of different components integrated into how we think, feel, and what we prioritize. Usually, we don't prioritize ourselves, which is why people tend to "let go of themselves." Considering that it's also much easier to quit or choose the easy route, rather than spending time looking after ourselves, preparing meals or getting active and moving our bodies as it was designed to do, it's clear that shifting your mind is the answer. Even though losing weight or changing your daily routine, waking up earlier, feeding your body the right foods, etc., seems like a lot of obstacles placed in your way, it's really just all in your mind.

That is why the best practice you could ever engage in starts with overcoming barriers in your mind, and, ultimately, taking control of it. It's not rocket science, and when you're in it, you'll discover that if you affirm a new idea of what you'd like to be or have in your life, you will obtain it.

Hypnosis is focused on pattern interruption or simply meeting the roots of patterns, and adjusting the factors that cause bad habits.

How to use hypnosis to change eating habits

1. Think yourself thin and implement affirmations to help you get there in a healthy and sustainable way by adopting the habits of people who have already reached their weight and body positivity goals.
2. Adjust your mind to assist your weight loss goals and support it every day.
3. Don't eat without thinking, which includes both emotional eating, binge eating, or any act of mindless eating. Recognize the differences between emotional eating and eating because you are hungry.
4. Enjoy cooking, and fill your home with good food instead of anything tempting. This will also help you to develop more controlled eating patterns. By not filling your home with sugary or fatty foods, you're instantly making a change. Although it's difficult, it's a bold one to be proud of.
5. Don't eat because of comfort; that usually leads to the over-consumption of calories.
6. Don't be reckless. If you're going to spend most of your time sitting in front of a television binge-watching your favorite series, you're bound to want to snack. Stay true to your affirmations and believes during hypnosis, and remind yourself to stay active throughout the day. This will prevent eating out of boredom and potentially lead to more weight-loss.
7. Stay motivated throughout your journey with hypnosis. Remembering that you're not going to achieve results overnight, but in the long haul, it is the answer to keeping both your mind and body in check.

How to conduct hypnosis the right way

Self-hypnotization can do wonders for your health and may also sound far too good to be true. However, many experts believe that changing our thought processes can lead to a much better state of health and quality of life.

To prepare yourself for this practice, you should:

- Focus on now instead of thinking about tomorrow

The future will always exist, but it's not something we can control, is it? Sure, we can control most things that influence it and builds up to it, but we cannot control much else. Often, the things we want and hope for, or even work for, don't always reflect back to us along the line or according to our planned timeline. Given that we are not in control of what lies ahead, there's no need to be worried about it. Giving the wrong things too much energy without knowing where it's going will instill the idea into our minds that we are not in control of our life. On that note, unless you're in control, can you really thrive? Can you really focus on the present? In essence, can you be happy or reach your goals? Thinking in this sense also translates in the context of today. Should you start on Monday–a day that is idealized as the perfect day to start something challenging or should you just start today, the day you can control?

- Jump into reality

The average human is extremely fixated on overthinking, and this is something that we don't necessarily feel like we have any control over. However, thinking about overcoming the habit of thinking too much may not even feel reasonable to some. Given that people who overthink are also considered much more emotional than others, hypnosis for weight loss can help individuals to overcome more than just bad habits related to their diet and lifestyle. It can also help them overcome the habit of overthinking a workout, planning too much, as well as obsessing over their calorie intake. With hypnosis, you will be able to rid your mind of overthinking processes and make healthier choices, which can get you a lot farther than thinking about everything you want, or still need to do. Finally, focusing on how your body feels when it's moving or even how it feels when it's consuming the right nutrients will trick your mind in wanting to implement change that will beneficially serve your body.

Detox your emotional state of mind

Anyone who is overweight, suffering from obesity or other eating disorders, is bound to have some type of emotional issue. Call it an emotional barrier, but it is something that holds most people back from losing weight. People don't struggle with weight loss because they are necessarily unaware of what to do. In fact, they may even know exactly what it is they must do but convince themselves that they can't get themselves to do it because of underlying emotional issues, which also translates into excuses and bad habits. Professional therapists will often prescribe their clients to feel their feelings instead of just supresing it. Once you feel and embrace it, you can finally make use of it and let it go. This will, in return, set your body up for success as you will be able to focus on what's good for you instead of holding on to what's not.

Implement powerful breathing techniques

Integrating powerful breathing, including diaphragmatic breathing is wonderful for amplifying your focus. When we focus on deep or controlled breathing, both our minds and bodies enter a state of being calm, allowing us to feel like we are in control. This also opens the door to feeling happier, allowing us to implement more positive habits and experiences into our days, rather than just going through a motion rut. Focusing on diaphragmatic breathing causes you to breathe deeply, which when you breath out, tightens and flattens your stomach. This not only relaxes your body but also creates the idea of visualization that you can indeed have a flat stomach.

Apart from diaphragmatic breathing, you should also try out Buteyko breathing. This type of breathing involves breathing small quantities of fresh air in and out of your nose, which reduces the total amount of oxygen you use. Given that most individuals over-breathe, they can't control their bodies when they are stressed. This contributes to bad digestion, inadequate sleeping patterns, and many other negative habits that contribute to weight gain. Implementing this breathing technique can solve one issue you struggle with but can translate into solving countless other issues you face. It will also reduce anxiety and place you in a more mindful state of living.

Chapter 3:

A basic self-hypnosis session for weight loss

Next, we will look at the art of manipulating your conscious and rewiring your subconscious to lose weight with the following six steps.

Step 1: Study or adjust your schedule to find time when you won't be distracted by your surroundings. This is a time set out for yourself where you are required to focus for 30 to 60 minutes to allow yourself to enter a trance state of mind where you feel completely relaxed and content without any interruptions.

Step 2: Set a weight loss intention to reach your goals, but rather than only focusing on how much weight you want to lose, focus on all the benefits that you will reap because of it. Since a weight loss journey is also considered to be a positive and reconstructive journey, make certain you allow space for focusing on the value you place on your body. Placing value on our bodies is extremely important and helpful. It can teach us respect and motivate a greater reason behind perseverance to complete what we set out to do. Visualizing how much weight you'd like to lose in a reasonable period will set the tone for your goal before you begin. Make sure you say your goal out loud to ensure that your intention is set.

Step 3: Visualize your end-goal. What does your body look like and what size are you? How do you feel once you get closer to your goal? Also focus on how you feel once you've reached your goal. Do you feel fulfilled and accomplished? Focus on the benefits you will reap once you've reached your goal, as well as the possibilities that will follow.

Step 4: Look the part. Close your eyes and enter a state of relaxation. Much like with meditation, your mind must be quiet and calm. Now you can engage in deep breathing for up to three minutes and choose your breathing technique, either the diaphragmatic technique or the Buteyko breathing technique. Make sure you continue to breathe until you feel calm and relaxed throughout your entire body. Now relax your body, you've entered a trance state of mind.

Step 5: Visualize yourself reaching your goal in a trance state of mind. How good do you feel in your skin now that you've reached your goal weight? Do you miss your bad habits, and do you feel better now that you've left them behind? Do people look up to you for losing weight? Focus on the positivity surrounding the fact that you've accomplished something you possibly didn't think was possible before. Continuing with this state of mind will allow you to change your behavior and increase the desire for you to implement change into your life.

Step 6: Return to your present state with ease, and don't rush it. You are in a relaxed state of mind and you should focus on bringing the feelings back to your reality. By doing this session daily and reminding yourself of how you feel, you will be able to adjust your mindset and increase the possibility of losing weight. You will receive new energy for taking on obstacles in your life and be able to make behavioral modifications where it is necessary.

Why weight loss hypnotherapy is for you

Have you ever thought about food as your friend?

Have you ever thought about your friends and family as a priority?

If you answer both of these questions honestly, you'll come to find that food is supposed to be your friend. Thinking of it in that way, you will surely treat it with more respect. Given that we only get one body and that our bill of health deteriorates over time, we are most definitely obliged to look after ourselves. The same goes for kicking bad habits like smoking, consuming too much alcohol, possibly consuming mind-altering drugs, and even other negative factors like depriving yourself of sleep.

Hypnosis is all about bettering yourself, and if you can reach a state where you are focused on improving your health and feel willing to do so daily, you will finally change your mindset toward food, exercise, and bad habits.

Eating food that is beneficial for your health will become second nature.

Setting an attainable goal for yourself, like reaching 21-days of eating clean, will eventually lead to everything that follows thereafter if you manage to stick to self-hypnosis. Twenty-one days of consistency will allow you to create new habits and familiarities, which will keep you on track even after you've reached your weight loss goals. After a while, eating healthily won't feel like a punishment, but rather like a reward.

You will feel better by eating better, but also eating less

If you're like most people, you probably love eating and food in general, right? Just because you follow a diet and workout routine, does not mean that you can't enjoy your food. However, keeping in mind that you have three meals a day, and possibly one or two snacks, you should be mindful that your body doesn't need too much food. If our stomach is the size of your two hands clasped together in a fist, then where does the rest of the food you consume go? It gets deposited as fat storage in your body, which is exactly what you don't want. Focus on mindful eating and listen to your body. You will also find that eating less actually satisfy you more.

It shifts your attitude tremendously

One of the biggest changes hypnosis implements is your mindset toward eating and exercising. While many individuals who engage in hypnosis do it to control their eating habits, there's a lot of change to be made to most people's sedentary lifestyles.

You are a human and you are designed to move, to hunt, to gather.

If you sit down all day and don't push your body out of its comfort zone, it will waste away and die.

Chapter 4: Hypnosis portion control session

Habits rule our lives and not only shape our current reality, but it also shapes our future reality.

Portion control is considered one of the biggest reasons why people gain weight, and although it may not make sense to some, it's truly something that can make or break your weight loss journey.

During hypnotherapy, you want to be in control of your mind, which will allow you to control your habits and tendencies you have with ease. There are many reasons why people overeat. Some may not even say that people make the decision to do so, which means it's also considered unmindful eating.

Is portion control difficult to maintain?

Yes, if you're not mindful about what you put in your mouth. If you've ever heard about the saying, "Too much of anything is not good for you," you should know by now that it's the truth, right?

After you've eaten something small or a large meal, you should ask yourself, "How did that meal make me feel? Does my body appreciate it, and will it benefit me in any possible way other than ensuring I'm full?"

Buffet meals at restaurants have become a popular occurrence. Just why do people feel the need to eat as much as they do?

Most therapists would emphasize the fact that their clients and people, in general, have underlying issues that result in bad habits, like overeating, to either forget or overcome emotional baggage, feelings, and unresolved issues.

It doesn't matter what your reasons may be, overeating is not considered healthy, and apart from causing your body to gain weight, it can affect your body negatively. It can also contribute to health issues, which can be recognized with symptoms, such as indigestion, feeling uncomfortably full regularly, water retention, and higher than average visceral fat in the abdominal region.

Needless to say, habits are in control of our lives, and we are more prone to overeating than we'd like to admit. The U.S. is the perfect example of a country that has created a culture around normalizing portions that are far too large for a person to consume. However, it is the norm and has contributed to over half of the country's residents suffering from either obesity or being overweight.

What people need to understand is that obesity isn't considered a body type. It is considered a severe health problem that can cause countless other health issues. These health issues include heart disease, stroke, diabetes, high blood pressure, cancer, gallbladder disease, gallstones, gout, osteoarthritis and breathing difficulties, including sleep apnea and asthma.

The reason why portion control is considered difficult is that we eat for all the wrong reasons.

Society is prone to gravitate toward foods that have an unbalanced level of sugar, sodium, unhealthy fats, and caloric content. These foods are also branded more appealing and are promoted wherever we feast our eyes accordingly. People are also used to overeating and have come to adopt it as a bad habit they can't seem to get rid of. Often people also convince themselves that they either can't waste food or feel forced to finish whatever they have on their plate. Other than that, overeating has become perceived as normal. Given that people are more bored, depressed or emotionally disrupted than ever before, including lazy, eating whatever they can find or opting for the bad option always seem like the best option.

Portion control plays a very important role in our well-being, as it can differentiate us from being healthy or unhealthy. It affects our bodies contributing to how much we weigh and makes us hold on to excess weight. If

you're following some type of 'healthy' diet and a reasonable workout routine, always go back and check whether you're eating either enough or too much, and if you are being mindful of your eating habits.

Controlling your portions doesn't only account for a slimmer body, but it also gives you more energy and boosts your metabolism. The more food you feed your body, the harder it must work to digest it, which is also why you may feel sluggish and lazy after overeating. Increased food consumption takes a lot more energy and may cause your metabolism to slow down as a means of defending itself against harm.

Hypnosis helps you to rediscover balance concerning your eating habits, allowing you to become in tune with and focused on your goals. In this way, you will also regain your self-worth, which may have become lost, along with your self-confidence and growth. You can attain all this and more by committing to hypnosis.

Taking it one step further, hypnosis is also thought to be much more effective for weight loss and any type of mind-body commitment, as it has been proven to have a success rate of up to 93% compared to other types of therapy (Meridian Peak Hypnosis, n.d.).

That statistic alone should make anyone want to give hypnosis integrated with food control a try.

Although many diet and workout routines are being sold online, some of which are even made available for free, the right approach for losing weight starts with your mind. Hypnosis offers a means of sustainable weight loss that provides us with access to our unconscious mind, eliminates any barriers and replaces it with thoughts that prove to be more helpful than any type of information. Hypnosis also allows us to dig deep into our minds, almost like we're exploring the files on our computers, and get rid of any negative associations we may have with developing new habits.

How to overcome portion control and overeating difficulties

We all need food to survive, but when does needing food get to a point where it results in overeating and overindulging? When is it necessary to check yourself, take a step back and stop eating?

Everyone who has an unhealthy relationship with food views it similarly. It often serves as a means of comfort and security that allows us to convince ourselves that it is acceptable to consume food recklessly and without thinking. Needless to say, unless you are trained in nutrition or pride yourself in the idea of

caring for your well-being, you probably don't have a very positive relationship with food.

If you've recognized the need to build a better relationship with food, and you would like to discover more about hypnosis for weight loss and to kick your bad habits, you have to identify the initial cause contributing to your problem. Since eating presents itself as a form of temporary stress-relief and distracts us from feeling emotions like stress, sadness, anxiety and anger, it's something we tend to gravitate toward at least at some point in our lives. Given that advertising companies are experts at presenting society with flawed foods that may seem appealing or are covered in somewhat "dietary-friendly" content, we have adopted the belief that it is okay to consume artificial food or whatever advertising suggests to us. We have equally taught ourselves that consuming unhealthy food acts as a reward for whatever we're doing right. For instance, telling yourself that you can eat whatever you want over the weekend after five weekdays of clean eating is entirely wrong. We should not be feeling like we are punishing ourselves by eating a healthy, balanced diet. It should become second nature to us as we adopt a healthy lifestyle.

The first step to using hypnosis for weight loss successfully is identifying the reasons why you struggle to achieve whatever it is you want. When undergoing self-hypnosis, you must learn how to address your food addiction and turn it into something useful, such as motivation to not feel as weak or inefficient as you do at your current weight or state of health. Before you start with your session, you should acknowledge the reason why your goal seems so out of reach, as well as what it is that's holding you back from achieving it.

During a professional hypnotherapy session, a therapist will generally ask you a list of questions related to weight loss, including questions about your diet and exercise habits. Since you are conducting the therapy session on your own, you can simply go over your daily routine and habits. Sometimes, it helps to write down both your positive and negative habits to see where it is you need to improve. You need to layout all of the information in front of you and focus on what it is you need to improve during your session. Writing down your goals will also help you to develop a clearer picture of where it is you'd like to go. Keep in mind that self-hypnosis is entirely up to you, so you have to commit and stay disciplined throughout the 21 days.

This period is attainable to most individuals and sets a benchmark for

yourself without having to make a commitment that is too big.

Since you have to reframe your food addiction, it's important to be honest about bad habits with yourself, which could include anything from binge eating, emotional eating, overeating or tricking yourself to believe that you need more food or most commonly used as an excuse, telling yourself that you'll start a diet on Monday.

Gathering the necessary information about yourself and your habits will help you discover what you need to correct and focus on.

Engaging in hypnotherapy, you will be able to improve your confidence through positive suggestions set out to make you feel empowered, reinvent your inner voice, which will remind you to keep a positive and healthy mindset, visualize yourself achieving your weight loss goals, identify unconscious patterns that led to your current unhealthy lifestyle, as well as get rid of any fear you may have in achieving your goals.

You probably didn't know that you could live in fear of achieving your goals. It sounds ridiculous, but changing yourself or the way you live could present itself as stressful too. Often people don't achieve their goals because they are fearful of leaving their comfort zone. Since we cannot thrive or grow without being uncomfortable in life, it's necessary to overcome such fears. Hypnosis will address your habit patterns and allow you to remove it from your subconscious. It will allow you to develop new and sustainable coping mechanisms. For example, with hypnosis, you can visualize yourself responding to a stressful interaction or situation and choose how you would like to react healthily manner. You will also imagine yourself eating healthy during the session to help you make better choices and form permanent eating habits.

To those who don't struggle with portion and craving control find it simple to stick to their routine way of eating. Compared to someone who is compulsive and eats based on their feelings, hypnosis is probably the best method of self-development. It works by controlling reactions and tendencies, which has obviously led to your pitfalls and unhealthy relationship with food. During the hypnosis session, you are recommended to find a way to dispatch your food cravings and eliminate bad habits surrounding portion control. This helps you visualize yourself having a much healthier relationship with food, which will set you up for success.

With hypnosis, it seems silly to just focus on physically losing weight. There are so many other factors involved that attributes to what causes weight gain

that you can rectify. Losing weight and achieving any health-related goal is a journey that will set you on a path to living your best life.

How to eat the right amount of food

To regain proper portion control and eat the right amount of food at each meal, you need to focus on eating the right types of food. Only then will you be able to maintain a balanced diet. It's always helpful to conduct a little research before you start with hypnosis, especially if your goal is to learn how to reduce your portion sizes and stick to it. Although you know the reasons why you should, and that eating too much food contributes to the unnecessary deposit of fat that gets stored in your body, a lot of people still overeat regardless. It's important to remind yourself that you shouldn't be living to eat, but rather eat to live. Once you've established this rule, you can control your portion sizes, and, ultimately, lose weight.

If you practice hypnosis or are already following a diet and you're not losing weight, then you probably have to evaluate your portion sizes. You also have to listen to your body and learn whether the type of food you're consuming is serving your body well. Carrying excess weight could be a result of overeating at meals. Also, overeating too frequently is the same as eating a bad diet; it's not good for your overall health or your weight loss journey.

Proper portion control alone won't make you lose all the weight, but it will give you more energy, particularly because constantly being full places strain on our bodily processes to work harder. This includes your metabolism, which if not working efficiently, could cause you to hold onto excess weight, completely halt your weight loss results, and cause you to feel uncomfortable. Having a weak metabolism and inadequate digestion could pose as a serious health issue and include disruptive symptoms, such as chronic fatigue, weight gain, depression, headaches, constipation, and sugar cravings.

The term "portion control," refers to eating an adequate amount of food. The quantity of what you consume, along with the type thereof, is required if your goal is weight loss. Often, people force themselves to finish the food on their plate out of politeness or because we can't seem to recognize that we've had enough.

To control your portion sizes, you can try doing the following:

- Eat slowly and be more conscious about what you eat.
- Drink a glass of water 15 minutes before you eat. This will fill your stomach and prevent you from eating too much in one sitting.
- Avoid buffets or eating 2-for-1 deals at restaurants.
- Use a smaller plate.
- Take photos of your meals and save them in a folder so that you can revisit and compare the size of your meals visually. This will also help you stay on track and keep improving.

Why hypnosis works for portion control

You can implement the above-mentioned methods for controlling your portion sizes at meals, but you still need to find a way to overcome bad habits. Eating compulsively is nothing to be proud of, and food must be considered as fuel. Improving the quality of your food often helps with portion control and can assist you in making the right decisions. Let's be real, nobody wants to eat a big plate of broccoli. Focusing on how eating small versus large quantities of food makes you feel will also help you to overcome any mental relation or need you may have to consume the right portions of food.

Once you manage to overcome your struggles with portion control, you will reach a deeply relaxed state of mind and feel empowered, as you won't feel like you have to overcome your unconscious any longer. You will now finally be in control.

Overcoming portion control is a massive challenge, yet it is not something that cannot be achieved. It is especially difficult to achieve in society today. What used to be regarded as proper portion sizes, have now doubled in the past 50 years. Since there is a new generation of people, it has also been normalized, which has been one of the main contributions to increased cases of obesity.

To fix any problem you may have related to consuming too many calories a day, whether it's overeating or eating empty calories, you must engage in mindfulness. This is something that can only be taught by yourself. It is not a skill, but rather an act of taking a step back and acknowledging what you are doing, for instance, what you are consuming, including the quantity thereof.

Hypnosis for portion control session

In this hypnosis for portion control session, we will be focused on six factors to integrate into your daily life, which will help you make better decisions regarding food choices, as well as the quantity of food you consume. While the goal of this hypnosis session isn't specifically focused on losing weight, but rather in eating less, learning how to control your portions will speed up your

metabolism and overall help you experience a better quality of life.

During this session, the six factors we will be focused on include:

1. Focus on eating smart - You will learn how to incorporate a different style of eating that is focused on decreasing your appetite and speeding up your metabolism. This initiative is focused on you eating six small meals per day, which includes a balance of carbohydrates, protein and vegetables. In this session, you will be focused on creating what you regard as being the perfect day in your mind, in which you imagine yourself eating smaller portions at meals.

2. Focus on shrinking your stomach - Integrating deep breathing into your hypnosis for portion control session, you will be focused on imagining having a small stomach. When you breathe in, you will imagine yourself as having a smaller, flatter stomach. Given that you prefer this image over your current look, you will be able to trick your brain to think that you prefer this version of yourself.

3. Focus on eating slowly - Control your cravings, including sugar and fast-food cravings, as well as eating too much at one sitting. This

can be done by imagining a timeline in which you finish your snack or meal. You shouldn't be rushing eating. By focusing on eating slowly, will be able to minimize your cravings.

4. Focus on drinking water - Serving as one of the most helpful tools to reduce cravings and overeating, drinking water to fill up your stomach will play a significant role in helping you overcome portion control. Since drinking water will also help you get rid of ailments, such as stress, fatigue, inflammation, digestive issues and depression, it will serve you far better than just eating yourself full.

5. Focus on greens and vegetables - When you're consuming too much food, the chances are that you are eating the wrong types of food. As I suggested previously, no one wants to eat a big serving of vegetables. That is why filling your plate with 50% of vegetables and leafy greens is a really good idea to help you imagine that you are still eating enough food visually. You can eat a salad the size of a regular plate for lunch, but you can't eat a plate of fries the size of a dinner plate for lunch. Plus, once you incorporate healthy eating into your daily routine, you won't want to eat as much food

because you will learn the value thereof.

6. Focus on the feeling of hunger - During your hypnosis session for portion control, you must acknowledge hunger. If you're not hungry, then you shouldn't be eating, and if you feel like you shouldn't be hungry because you ate a little while ago, drink a glass of water before turning to food. When you are hungry, however, focus on what your body needs and not what is either convenient or tastes better than a healthier option. Finding foods that are healthy to integrate into your daily diet is also very helpful and important. It could make the difference between whether or not you stick to a healthy eating plan.

Session:

This hypnosis session will have a deeply relaxing effect on you, and that is why you shouldn't be listening to this while driving, operating machinery, or looking after anyone else. If you need to awaken for any reason, you will do so easily and become comfortably alert. It's also okay if you fall asleep. Your subconscious mind will continue to listen to my voice, and you will still benefit from this hypnosis session.

Hypnosis is very relaxing. It's safe and positive, and you are always completely and fully in control. Just trust in yourself, relax, and enjoy the experience.

So now, find a quiet and comfortable place, either sitting or lying down with your head supported. Find a place where you know you won't be disturbed, where you can remain for the duration of this hypnosis session, and we'll get started.

Now that you find yourself in a quiet and comfortable position, arms resting by your sides, legs uncrossed, let us begin to absorb ourselves in relaxation and calmness. This is a time to be as lazy as you want, to let yourself go, and to allow yourself to become deeply relaxed. So, begin relaxing now. Let the muscles soften. With the next exhalation, drop the shoulders, and allow the body to sink into the surface below. Beginning to let go of everything, all thoughts, all tensions, and tightness. Let go of everything and become deeply soothed, deeply calm, and deeply relaxed. Listening quietly to the sound of my voice, any other sounds you may hear will fade into the distance. My voice will guide you with the deepest level of relaxation, including the mind and the body.

All you need to do is let go. Let go, and follow the suggestions I make. All of the suggestions I make are here to benefit you. If your eyes are not already closed, do so gently now.

Take a long, slow, and steady breath in, all the way down into the stomach. Hold the breath for a moment, and breathe out slow and steady. Focusing completely on the breath, letting go, and now relaxing a little more with each exhalation. Take another long, slow, and steady breath in all the way down to the bottom of the stomach. This time, hold the breath for a moment longer, and breathing out, all the way out slowly and steadily, letting go of everything. Letting the shoulders drop a little as the muscles may go, softening any tension or tightness in the body. Take one slow and steady breath all the way down to the bottom of the stomach, holding the breath a moment longer again and breathing all the way out, feeling more centered, calmer, steadier, continuing to relax a little further and more deeply with every exhalation. While you're continuing with your deep, steady, relaxing, breathing, notice the eyelids. As you peek through the eyelids, what colors do you see reflecting back?

Is there a dominant color? Does the color move? Perhaps it swirls or flickers, or even takes certain shapes. Or does the color remain still? Stay with this for a moment. Hold the gaze. Become comfortable in the feeling, allow the feeling to soften and let it provide comfort. Let the comfort deepen, just focusing on the color. Gazing at the color, notice how the color creates a stillness within. Let any thoughts or interruptions move through the mind. Move through the mind, or even floating up and out of it. You are safe, you are special, you are calm, you are becoming even more calm with every slow and steady breath you take.

In a moment, I'm going to count down from five to one, and when I get to one, you will have relaxed all the way down to a deep and comfortable space.

5 - Deepen now that feeling of relaxation. Feeling a gentle warmth touching the skin, a calm and comfortable warmth that will spread down slowly from the top of the head to the tips of the toes. As that subtle sensation of warmth moves down through the body, every sound, every muscle that it touches, relaxes and unwinds. Beginning now at the top of the head, and feeling now as the relaxation spreads down, down through the scalp, across the forehead, the muscles of the forehead softening, flattening and letting go, you may even feel a gentle tingling in the scalp and forehead as the relaxation moves down and throughout. Letting that gentle warmth spread down the face, down over the eyes, down the sides of the face, and letting go. Feel the comfortable warmth and relaxation spreading, spreading farther down over the nose, the top lip, and now the bottom lip, down into the jaw, allowing the muscles in the jaw to soften, feeling it relaxing and letting go, more deeply relaxed. The whole head now feels relaxed, sinking farther down and drifting, floating.

4- As all the muscles in the head continue to relax even more, feel that gentle tingling, warmth and relaxation, moving down into the neck, through the back of the neck, the sides of the neck, and the front of the neck. Letting that relaxation spread down now, down into the shoulders, deep into the muscles of the shoulders, the fibers all letting go. Letting go just like an elastic band being released, moving into a relaxed and loose state. All tension and tightness decipitating. Your relaxation and calmness spreading down to the arms, through the biceps and triceps, to the elbows, the forearms, and down through the hands to the tips of the fingers. Allow the arms to simply let go. Let them sink more deeply down, noticing how they feel more relaxed and lighter. Noticing just how they feel with deep relaxation moving all the way down and through them.

3 - You can feel that calmness now, spreading down through the body. Now feeling that deep relaxation is ready to spread down all through the back. Beginning now, at the base of the neck, allowing relaxation to move slowly and deeply down through the back one vertebrae at a time. Allowing the

vertebrae to let go of any tension, feeling the whole of the back now, letting go. Letting go, and sinking down, down to the deepest level of relaxation, drifting and floating.

2 - Everything relaxing, everything feeling loose and heavy, feeling the calmness and comfort through the hips and thighs now moving down through the knees. Down, through the hips and shins. A relaxation spreading down through the foot, the sole of the foot, down into the toes. It is going down and down, drifting and floating more and more deeply relaxed.

1 - Everything feeling loose, heavy, light, relaxed. The whole body now feeling so relaxed, so heavily relaxed that even if you wanted to move an arm or leg it would take way too much energy to do so. You can enjoy this feeling of deep relaxation, and letting go. You can enjoy it again, and again, and again, every time you listen to this deep relaxation. Every time you listen to my voice, and the words that I say, your body will instinctively follow the requests to relax, and it will relax more intently, more deeply each and every time. The more you relax, the more you can relax. Now that you are enjoying this peace and relaxation, your mind is interested and ready to welcome these positive and beneficial words that I say.

As you are relaxing, now, take a moment to congratulate yourself on this wonderful journey that you're on. Give yourself a pat on the back because you're doing great. You're doing great because you've taken the first step. You've already taken the step to start. You've started, which is well beyond the point where many people have stopped. It's hard to believe, isn't it? However, many people don't get this far, unfortunately for them. These people won't ever see a positive change in themselves. Nothing is going to change when they keep on doing the same old things. You know that because you're different, and because you're different, you're already changing. You're doing a mind-shift, and a physical shift is about to come. You've managed to move forward. You're empowering yourself right now, just by getting started. You're listening to this progressive hypnosis program, and you do know that now that you've started, there's no turning back.

You're not a quitter.

You're in this for the long haul.

You want this.

You really want this.

You're ready and committed, and this is your time, your health, and your pride.

So, it's important to know why you want this, and I mean really know. What's your reason for wanting to become slimmer? Do you want to become healthier? Do you need to improve your health? Will being slimmer improve your posture, remove aches and pains? Do you want to be around longer for the sake of your family? Do you have special people in your life who can't afford to lose you? Do you want to walk into a clothing store and buy them off the rack? Do you want to return to a previous smaller size?

Do you want to wear clothes that increase your confidence and imitate your style instead of bigger and baggy clothes?

What is the most important reason to you for becoming slimmer? The answer will come to you instantly. Lock it in now.

Now, create a picture of yourself, your ideal size and shape, full of energy and health, an abundance of confidence. Make the picture bright and shiny. See yourself happy and content. Highlight the most important reason you have for becoming slimmer. See yourself wherever you need to be, and see yourself doing it well with ease, confidently. Let the pressure of doing this well within you. Let it grow and deepen. Keep increasing it, take it to a higher level, and let it swell around you.

Harness that feeling. Lock that feeling in now. Every time you are presented with a choice to not be healthy, return back to that feeling. Return your subconscious mind back to a picture that reminds you of your decision to be healthier, along with your reasons that support it.

By doing this, you will easily make the right choices, each and every time you are presented with a challenge. This change is a must for you. If you don't make the change now, will you ever? If you keep doing things the same way, you will always get the same things. Action equals change, and you are committed to action.

How will it feel when you reach your ultimate size and shape?

How will it feel? It will feel fantastic, uplifting, rewarding, empowering. You'll be able to reach new heights in everything you try. The world will be your oyster. You'll be capable of anything you put your mind to. You have the power to become the ultimate you. Let your mind drift out, drift out into the future a few months from now. Find yourself walking past a familiar shopping strip. As you walk along the shopping strip, you catch a glimpse of a figure in the window you're walking past. The figure is walking along the strip just as you are. Their gage is purposeful, shoulders back, head high, posture strong and confident. They exude self-worth and energy, their figure lean and fit. You stop and turn to look at the figure front on, and you find the figure looking straight back at you.

Then you realize, it is you staring back. You are staring at your reflection. You are looking at your ultimate self, admiring your size and shape. You are fit, you are strong, and exuding energy and confidence. You are poised and in control, proud. You are aware of just how good it feels to feel this way. You reach out toward the glass, just as your reflection does, and when you touch your fingers to the glass, you realize your touch reflecting. You feel the energy bolt through your body and snap your attention, standing up straighter and taller.

You know exactly what to do to reach your ultimate shape and health. You've known it all this time, but it was buried. It's clear now. You now know how to make it happen. Now that you are aware of what to do, confidence and excitement glow within you. You are now, finally, back in charge of your life. This is the real you. This is the way you were born to be, born to look, and feel. You are slim, healthy, happy, fit, in charge, and confident.

Each and every day. With each and every food choice and portion size, you are moving closer to your ultimate weight, closer to the ultimate you. You

feel and look fabulous, and it's all because you're thriving on a journey to become the ultimate you. All these great changes are taking place within you at a deep, subconscious level. Every day you are stronger, more determined, and have more enthusiasm for everyone and everything around you. Now, all of these suggestions are firmly embedded in your subconscious mind and grow stronger and stronger every day.

In a moment, I will count up from one to five, and when I reach the number five, you will be wide awake, fully alert and refreshed. You will be ready to allow these suggestions to work for you.

1 - Coming slowly back, taking some time to remember the pleasant feelings that you felt, aware of my voice, the comfort of your body.

2 - Becoming more and more awake, the energy-returning back into your body in the present moment.

3 - Letting the energy spread through your entire body again, your arms, your legs your feet, and your head, all the energy restoring back to normal.

4 - Stretching out fully now, wiggling your fingers and toes, eyelids, beginning to flutter. Take a deep, reenergizing breath in, just like after taking a long, restful sleep.

5 - Wide awake now. Eyes open wide and fully alert, mind and body fully awake, feeling really good and looking forward to the rest of your day.

More than 100 affirmations to reach your fitness goals

The following affirmations will help you to reach your fitness goals. Replay these whenever you feel the need to reaffirm for affirmations. They will help you to accomplish your weight loss goals and get the most from hypnosis.

- I have a fast metabolism.
- I am living a healthy lifestyle.
- It is really easy for me to lose weight.
- I am attaining and maintaining my desire to wait.
- I love exercising.
- I love working out.
- I love eating natural, organic food.
- I am now creating healthy eating habits.
- I have a strong urge to only eat healthy foods.
- I find it easy to stay in shape.
- I am closer and closer to my ideal weight.
- My body is slim, healthy, and strong.
- Every day, in every way, I am getting slimmer and fitter.
- I often visualize myself in my ideal weight.

- I burn calories easily and frequently.
- I love myself unconditionally.
- It is easy for me to control my weight.
- Losing weight is easy and fun.
- I can do this, I am doing this, and my body is losing weight right now.
- I love eating high-alkaline foods.
- I burn calories with every breath I take.
- I am grateful for my strong, fit body.
- My stomach is toned.
- My arms are toned.
- I am in shape.
- I am dedicated to staying in shape.
- I give myself full permission to lose weight and to be fit.
- I choose to drink alkaline water and stay hydrated.
- I enjoy eating fruits and vegetables.
- I am becoming lighter and stronger every day.
- Every day, in every way, I am getting better and better.
- I practice intermediate fasting, and it works.
- I exercise three or more times a week, and I love it.
- I believe in my ability to lose weight and keep it off.
- I am completely motivated to living a healthy and fit lifestyle.

- I am now experiencing my ideal weight.
- I believe in myself.
- I am ready to lose weight.
- I am thinner and thinner each moment.
- I have the power to change my life.
- My body becomes more attractive each day.
- I am in control of what I eat and drink.
- I respect my body enough to look after it.
- I am in control of my life.
- I will achieve my goals, and nothing will hold me back.
- I am in control of my weight loss journey.
- It's so easy to lose excess weight.
- I am burning fat right now.
- I am full of energy and thriving.
- I am creating a body that I like and enjoy, compared to my current body.
- I accept myself the way I am.
- I am ready to be healthy and attractive.
- Losing weight comes naturally to me.
- I choose to be the best version of myself that I can possibly be.
- I am stronger than any excuses I have bottled up previously.
- I make healthy choices for my body and well-being.
- I am self-reliant and persistent in everything I do every day.
- I look and feel great.
- I am now the perfect weight and the perfect size.
- I am open to positive changes in every area of my life.
- Whatever I conceive to believe, I will achieve.
- My body is free of unwanted emotions that contribute to weight gain.
- My body is free from unwanted emotions that keep my body from losing weight.
- I have all that I need to succeed.
- I am motivated.
- I am powerful.
- My behavior is aligned with my balanced state of mind.
- Everything that I do serves my goals without affecting others.
- Each day I completely trust my intuition.
- I am healthy.
- I am beautiful.
- I am wise.
- I am made with the purpose to achieve great things.
- I am the perfectly complete owner of my body.
- I am a magnet attracting abundance in my life.
- Fear is just a feeling. I overcome it and move on from it.
- I don't embrace fear.

- I am successful in any area of my life.
- I am polite and respectful to any person I meet.
- I am patient.
- I am the only one who can stop myself from losing weight.
- I am the only one who can make myself feel bad about the way I look.
- I am the only one who can convince myself that I am capable of whatever I put my mind to.
- I can lose weight and be happy.
- Once my sight is set on my goals, nothing can ever keep me from achieving it.
- Everything is good here right now.
- I trust that I am doing my best always.
- I am at peace with myself.
- I respect myself and I know that everything I do is meant to fulfill me.
- I am open-minded and will take advantage of any opportunities that surround me.
- All my relationships have a purpose and they fulfill me.
- I choose to see all the opportunities surrounding me.
- Prosperity surrounds and fulfills me.
- Prosperity flows toward me and through me.
- I can do amazing things.

- I am worthy.
- I am balanced.
- Everything that I need comes to me at the right moment.
- I am powerful and present in my own life.
- I have the power to take full control of my life.
- I am proud of who I am.
- I only want to improve my life.
- I want to move and be as active as I possibly can.
- I am special.
- I cannot change another person. I just let others be themselves, and I simply and solely accept myself.
- I am at ease with the uncontrollable things happening in my life.
- I am ready for any challenges that come my way.
- I focus on the good in any given situation.
- I am aware of my mistakes and I learn from them.
- I make good decisions.
- I appreciate everything surrounding me.
- I am calm and relaxed in any circumstances.
- I am the creator of my own life. I build its foundation, and I choose its content.
- I am filled with energy, and I exude happiness.

- I am far superior to negative thoughts and low actions.
- I am blessed with infinite talents and I use them every day.
- I peacefully detach myself from negative people every day.
- I am inspired with new and good ideas.
- I am content with all my accomplishments.
- I am brave and I am kind.
- I am a positive person and my life is filled with prosperity.
- I am admired and many people acknowledge my results.
- Compassion washes away my anger and replaces it with love.
- I am blessed with health and motivation.
- I am in control.
- I am at peace with everything that happened, happens, and will happen in my life.
- I am a wonderful human being.
- I am proud of everything I have accomplished so far.
- I feel good in my own skin.
- All the universe's beauty lies within me.
- I trust myself to create an amazing life.
- I am ambitious with my goals and plan to achieve them.
- I am fearless and I take risks.
- I accept new experiences.

- I am confident in everything that I do and believe in.
- I am curious and willing to learn new things.
- I am grateful for my life.
- I want to learn new skills and evolve.
- I am happy for other people and respect their work ethic.
- I profoundly love and respect myself.
- I am able to achieve great things in my life.
- I am comfortable being alone in my own company.
- My inner voice is always positive in any given situation.
- I reach all of my weight loss goals whenever I want.
- I completely trust myself.
- Positivity exudes from my mind.
- I can easily say no to something I know doesn't add value to my growth or life.
- I am persistent with my workout routine and eating habits.
- I choose to have a mindful relationship with food.
- I choose to have a mindful relationship with my body.
- I want to be active every day and stretch my body to avoid injuries.
- I am productive.
- I am in control of every aspect of my life.
- I am a hard worker.

- I find it easy to constantly work and be productive as much as I can.
- I don't engage in anything unnecessary or distracting to my work and goals.
- I am effective in my work daily.
- I am productive, motivated, and extremely hard-working.
- I create my own success.
- I attract abundance into my life.
- I always follow through on all of my plans.
- I am worthy of abundance in everything that I do.
- I wisely react to any challenge that comes my way.
- I believe in the power of positive thinking.
- I am a creator and a doer.
- I am important and know that I have a great deal of significance to offer this world.
- I am respected.
- I am filled with energy and determination.
- I am aware of my value, and I never allow others to bring me down.
- I can do anything I want.
- I am successful in all my actions.
- I am free to be myself.
- I am worthy to be loved and respected by a wonderful partner.
- I attract long-lasting friendships into my life.
- My mind can make wishes come true.
- I am humble and content in everything I do.
- I am always ready to learn.
- I forgive myself for any mistakes that I've made in the past.
- I react with love in any given situation.
- I am in control of everything that I think and do.
- I face any challenge I am presented with, with courage.
- I am loved.
- My life is abundant in health, wealth, and happiness.
- I accept everyone around me.
- I am a miracle.
- I am powerful.
- I am limitless.
- I am loving taking care of my temple, which is my body.
- Happiness is present wherever I go.
- Happiness is present in everything I shift my attention toward.
- My thoughts are positive.
- Each day is a gift that I gratefully accept.
- I am capable of building a bright future.
- My goals are real, and I can achieve them.
- I enjoy every process of making my dreams come true.
- I am kind and courageous.

- I heal myself from any frustration and anxiety.
- I am safe.
- The past is gone, and I only focus on the present.
- My personality exudes confidence.
- I am bold and outgoing.
- I am well-groomed, healthy, and full of confidence.
- My outer self is matched by my inner confidence and well-being.
- I have integrity.
- I am totally reliable and do what I say.
- I am surrounded by people who encourage me to be better every day.
- I support healthy choices instead of bad ones.
- I am in harmony with the night and the sleep that will come with it.
- I am safe, calm, and peaceful.
- All my deeds and thoughts are filled with love and kindness.
- I am organized and disciplined in everything I do.
- I am aware of how I feel, and it feels good.
- I bravely enter this world filled with endless possibilities and happiness.
- I am constantly learning.
- Wealth constantly comes into my life in many different forms.
- I let go of everything that is bothering me.
- I let go of poverty thinking and welcome abundance thinking.
- I am receptive to all the wealth life has to offer.
- I am the master of my existence.
- I am at peace with everything I do.
- I am able to achieve success with grace.
- I am extremely wealthy because I pursue all my dreams.
- I am deeply grateful for the wealth that keeps entering my life.
- There are no limits to the amount of wealth I can own.
- I become better and better with each passing day.
- I have the power to reach all my goals.
- I am kind, loving, and caring toward those who surround me.
- I am calm in every situation life presents me with.
- I have faith and trust in my intuition.
- I acknowledge my potential.
- I am worthy of health, positive energy, and calm.
- My world is filled with beauty and wealth.
- I am an amazing human being.
- I am a positive person with positive feelings for myself and for others.
- I am vibrating with energy and love.

- I have the power to create a beautiful life.
- I am a wonderful being, and I choose to love and respect myself.
- I learn from everything happening in my life, both of which are positive and negative.
- I am aware that mistakes are lessons, and I learn from each of them accordingly.
- I am determined to put in all my effort toward reaching my needs.
- I love and accept each thought and feeling.
- I reach out to everybody with love and empowerment.
- I am loved, and I am at peace with everything surrounding me.
- I am a creator of peace in my heart and in my soul.
- I choose to free myself from all fears and destructive doubts.
- I am at peace with myself and all the people surrounding me.
- I am open to love and happiness.
- I overcome every obstacle with ease and awareness.
- My life becomes greater and greater with each day that passes.
- I love and respect my body.
- I am worthy of everything that is good.
- I am a force to be reckoned with.
- I am a unique blend of love and power.
- I am healthy and energized.
- The universe loves me, supports me, and brings only positive experiences into my life.
- I am encouraged of all success that I achieve.
- I am blessed.
- I am constantly learning from my mistakes.
- I have everything that I need within me.
- I am happy with my age.
- I am enough for this moment I am in right now.
- All my relationships are in harmony, as my whole life is filled with appreciation and gratitude.
- I am beautiful on both the inside and outside.
- I am aware of my faults, and I choose to accept myself exactly as I am.
- I focus only on my life, and I let others live theirs.
- I am talented and special.
- I accept myself in all of my uniqueness.
- I don't accept negative thoughts and choose to replace it with positive ones.
- I don't accept negative energy and choose to replace it with affirmations.
- I take part in repetition to achieve sustainable goals.
- I love everything I see in me.

- I stay in the present and fully enjoy every moment of it.
- I am the creator of my own reality and completely in charge of may present.
- I am open to any change in my life.
- I am love, light, and happiness and my future is bright.
- I take care of my mind, my body, and my spirit.
- My flaws are beautiful, and I accept them in every form.
- Health, vitality, and happiness are constantly surrounding me.
- I am completely aware of my feelings, no matter the circumstances I am presented with.
- I deserve to be loved.
- I deserve to be respected and live a happy life.
- I am worthy.
- I am beautiful, and everybody respects me for who I am.
- I have value.
- I am motivated.
- I am consistent and disciplined in my work.
- I am in control of shaping my future.
- I trust my inner wisdom and my instincts.
- I am fully and completely loved by those surrounding me.
- Loving people are present in my life and they fill my day with optimism.
- I am marvelous.
- I am gracious.
- I am charming.
- I am kind.
- I am in control of my thoughts and feelings.
- I can shape new and positive habits whenever I want.
- I have a grateful heart that attracts what I deeply desire.
- The world is a wonderful place to be in, and I enjoy my enthusiastic journey living on this planet.
- I am surrounded with joy and peace everywhere I go.
- I am a creative and innovative human being.
- I am happy with the process of reaching my goals and doing what it takes to achieve it.
- I am patient in every activity I engage in.
- My body is healthy, and my mind is stable.
- My soul is at peace.
- I am talented and I use this gift every day.
- I forgive those who have hurt me, and I also forgive myself.
- I let go of the things I cannot control.
- I am a loving human being, and I am guided with courage every day.
- I overcome my fears successfully, even though they may seem difficult.

- I am brave, and therefore resilient.
- Creative energy surges through my mind and assists my dreams.
- I have endless opportunities waiting for me to grab hold of them.
- My mind overflows with ideas.
- In my mind, I can let go of my negative eating habits and implement new ones successfully.
- During my workouts, I can push myself to achieve what I want, no matter the pain I'm in.
- I accept where I am at the moment and choose to always improve my life, my wel-lbeing, and only focus on the things I can control in my life.

Chapter 5:

Hypnotic Gastric Band Techniques

There are many different types of hypnosis that benefits the human body in different ways. Some of these methods include hypnosis for weight loss and healthy living, which are different types of hypnosis for weight loss. Gastric band hypnotherapy is one of them and popularly known as a type of hypnotic state that is suggested to your subconscious, which involves fitting a gastric band around your stomach. This in return helps you lose weight, along with general hypnosis for weight loss sessions.

This type of hypnotherapy is often considered as the final type of hypnotherapy people try if they would like to reach their goals. The practice involves surgery known as gastric band surgery. During surgery, a gastric band gets fitted around the upper section of your stomach, with the purpose to limit the total amount of food you consume daily. This is a more extreme type of hypnotherapy for weight loss, which has proven to help people lose weight. Since it is surgical, you cannot carry out this method yourself. It also includes potential risks, which is why it must be treated with respect and only carried out by a certified medical practitioner.

You can, however, implement gastric band hypnotherapy yourself. It is a technique most commonly used by hypnotherapists with the purpose to trick the subconscious in believing that a gastric band has been fitted when in reality it hasn't. Since hypnotherapy is focused on putting your conscious mind on silent, and implementing thoughts and beliefs in your subconscious mind, as a type of hypnotherapy, it is quite effective. Given that hypnotherapy offers us many benefits, as well as allow us to imagine and come to terms with what we are capable of doing, it acts as the perfect solution to reaching some of your goals that may seem out of reach.

Gastric band hypnotherapy involves the process of believing that you have experienced the physical surgery itself, ultimately making you believe that the size of your stomach itself has been reduced too.

The gastric band used in gastric band fitting surgery is an adjustable silicone structure, used as a device to lose weight. This gastric band is used during surgery and placed strategically around the top section of your stomach, leaving a small space above the device. The space left open above the gastric band restricts the total amount of food that is stored inside the stomach. This is done to implement proper portion control every day and prevents overeating. The fitted gastric band physically makes it difficult for one to consume large amounts of food, which can set you in the habit of implementing proper portion control daily. This will essentially cause you to feel fuller after eating less, which in return encourages weight loss.

Most people choose to have the surgery after they've tried other methods to lose weight, including yo-yo dieting, diet supplements or over the counter drugs, all with the hope to lose weight. Gastric band surgery acts as a final resort for those who desperately want to lose weight and have been struggling for a long time.

Gastric band hypnotherapy serves as a very useful method as it can allow you to obtain a similar result as the gastric band fitting surgery itself. That's because you are literally visualizing getting the same procedure done and how you benefit from it. During gastric band hypnosis, you are visualizing yourself losing weight subconsciously, which translates into your conscious reality.

Hypnotherapists that specialize in gastric band hypnotherapy focus on finding the root of what prevents their clients from losing weight. Most of the time, they discover that emotional eating is one of the leading causes that contribute to people holding on to their weight. They also make a point of addressing experiences that remains in your subconscious mind but is yet to be addressed. These experiences often cause people to turn toward unmindful and emotional eating, which then develops into a pattern that feels impossible to kick.

Since stress is added to our lives every day, and people don't stop and take the time to process feelings or perhaps not even give it a thought, most turn to food for comfort. This also plays into emotional eating, which has extremely negative effects on the body long-term as it also contributes as one of the leading causes of obesity.

Given that obesity is an incredibly bad illness and more people get diagnosed with the condition every day, it is something that needs to be addressed. If gastric band hypnotherapy can prevent it or restructure our thinking patterns to not act on our emotions, but rather invite and process it, then it is a solution that everyone who needs to lose weight should try.

Once a hypnotherapist learns about why you're struggling to implement proper portion control, they will address it with the virtual gastric band treatment at a subconscious level. During this visualization session, you will have imagined that you have undergone the operation and had the gastric band placed around your upper stomach. This will lead you to think that you feel fuller quicker, serving as a safer options opposed to the surgery.

How gastric band hypnotherapy works

Hypnotherapy for weight loss, particularly for portion control, is great because it allows you to focus on creating a healthier version of yourself safely.

When gastric band fitted surgery gets recommended to people, usually because diets, weight loss supplements, and workout routines don't seem to work for them, they may become skeptical about getting the surgery done.

Nobody wants to undergo unnecessary surgery, and you shouldn't have to either. Just because you struggle to stick to a diet, workout routine or lack motivation, does not mean that an extreme procedure like surgery, is the only option. In fact, thinking that it is the only option you have left, is crazy.

Some hypnotherapists suggest that diets don't work at all. Well, if you're motivated and find it easy to stick to a diet plan and workout routine, then you should be fine. However, if you're suffering from obesity or overweight and don't have the necessary drive and motivation needed, then you're likely to fail. When people find the courage and determination to recognize that they need to lose weight or actually push

themselves to do it, but continuously fail, that's when they tend to give up.

Gastric band hypnotherapy uses relaxation techniques, which is designed to alter your way of thinking about the weight you need to lose, provides you a foundation to stand on and reach your goals, and also constantly reminds you of why you're indeed doing what you're doing. It is necessary to develop your way of thinking past where you're at in this current moment and evolve far beyond your expectations.

Diets are also more focused on temporary lifestyle changes rather than permanent and sustainable ones, which is why it isn't considered realistic at all. Unless you change your mind, you will always remain in a rut that involves first losing, and then possibly gaining weight back repeatedly. Some may even throw in the towel completely.

Since your mind is incredibly powerful, it will allow you to accept any ideas or suggestions made during your hypnosis gastric band hypnosis session. This can result in changing your behavior permanently as the ideas practiced during the session will translate into the reality of your conscious mind. By educating yourself on healthy habits, proper nutrition and exercise, you also stand a better chance of reaching your weight loss goals sustainably.

The gastric band fitting procedure will require a consultation with your hypnotherapist where you will discuss what it is you would like to gain from hypnotherapy. After establishing your current health status, positive and negative habits, lifestyle, daily struggles, and goals, they will recommend the duration of hypnotherapy you will require to see results. During this time, you need to inform your hypnotherapist of your diet and physical activity history. They are likely to ask you questions about your current lifestyle and whether you changed it over the years. If you've lived a healthy lifestyle before, then they will try to find and address the reasons why you let go of yourself and your health. If you have always lived your current unhealthy and unbalanced lifestyle, they will trace it back through the years with the hope to discover the reasons behind it. During your initial session, your weight loss attempts, eating habits, and any health issues you may experience will be addressed. Your attitude toward food will also be acknowledged, as well as your relationship with it, with people, and your surroundings.

Now your therapist will have a better idea of the type of treatment you need. The procedure is designed to have you experience the gastric band surgery subconsciously, as though it has really taken place. You will be talked to in a deep, relaxed state, exactly the same as standard hypnosis. During this session, you will be aware of everything happening around you. Suggestions to help boost your self-esteem and confidence are often also incorporated into the session, which can also assist you in what you would like to achieve consciously.

You will be taken through the procedure step-by-step. Your hypnotherapist may also make theater noises to convince your subconscious even more. After your session, your hypnotherapist may give you self-hypnosis guides and techniques to help you practice a similar session for the results to become more effective. Sometimes, gastric band hypnotherapy only requires a few sessions, depending on what your needs are.

Gastric band hypnosis doesn't only involve having to go to physical hypnotherapy sessions, but it also requires you to implement some type of weight management program that specifically addresses your nutrition, addiction, and exercise habits. It addresses habits between your body and mind and helps you implement new constructive ones.

After gastric band hypnosis, you can expect to feel as though you have a much healthier relationship with food, as well as a more mindful approach in everything you do. During the visualization process of gastric band fitting surgery, you will come to believe that your stomach has shrunk, which will trick your brain to think that you need less food. This will also make you think that you don't need a lot of food, which will make you more acquainted with consuming healthier portion sizes.

Gastric band hypnotherapy is successful as it makes you think that you are full after eating the daily recommended amount of food for your body. It is also considered much healthier than overeating or binge eating. You will learn to recognize the sensation of hunger versus being full, which will help you articulate between the two and cultivate healthier eating habits.

Hypnotherapy for different types of gastric banding types of surgeries

There are three types of gastric banding surgeries that could be used during hypnotherapy. These include:

- Sleeve Gastrectomy
- Vertical Banded Gastroplasty
- Mixed Surgery (Restrictive and Malabsorptive)

Gastric banding surgeries are used for weight loss. Depending on what your goal is with this weight-loss method, you can choose which option works best for you. The great thing about hypnotherapy with gastric band firming surgery is that

you can get similar results if you practice the session consistently.

During gastric banding surgery, the surgeon uses a laparoscopy technique that involves making small cuts in the stomach to place a silicone band around the top part of your stomach. This band is adjustable, leaving the stomach to form a pouch with an inch-wide outlet. After you've been banded in surgery your stomach can only hold one ounce of food at a time, which prevents you from eating more than you need to in one sitting. It also prevents you from getting hungry.

Given that it is an invasive procedure, most people don't opt for it as an option to lose weight. During the procedure, you are also placed under anesthesia, which always involves some risks. Nevertheless, the procedure has resulted in up to 45% of excess weight loss, which means that it can work for anyone looking to shed weight they are struggling to lose. The procedure can also be reversed should the patient not be happy with the effects thereof. When reversed, the stomach will return to the initial size it had before the surgery. (WebMD, n.d.)

Undergoing one of these three gastric banding surgeries, there are some side-effects involved, which includes the risk of death. However, this is only found in one of every 3000 patients. Other than that, common problems post-surgery include nausea and vomiting, which can be reduced by simply having a surgeon adjust the tightness of the gastric band.

Minor surgical complications, including wound infections and risks for minor bleeding, only occur in 10% of patients. (WebMD, n.d.)

As opposed to gastric bypass surgery, gastric banding doesn't prevent your body from absorbing food whatsoever, which means that you won't have to worry about experiencing any vitamin or mineral loss in your body.

Types of gastric banding techniques used in hypnotherapy for weight loss

- Sleeve gastrectomy - This procedure involves physically removing half of a patient's stomach to leave behind space, which is usually the size of a banana. When this part of the stomach is taken out, it cannot be reversed. This may seem like one of the most extreme types of gastric band surgeries, and due to its level of extremity, it also presents a lot of risks. When the reasons why the sleeve gastrectomy is done and gets reviewed, it may not seem worth it. However, it has become one of the most popular methods used in

surgery, as a restrictive means of reducing a patient's appetite. It is particularly helpful to those who suffer from obesity. It has a high success rate with very few complications, according to medical practitioners. Those who have had the surgery have experienced losing up to 50% of their total weight, which is quite a lot for someone suffering from obesity. It is equally helpful to those who suffer from compulsive eating disorders, like binge eating. When you have the procedure done, your surgeon will make either a very large or a few small incisions in the abdomen. The physical recovery of this procedure may take up to six weeks. (WebMD, n.d.)

- Vertical banded gastroplasty - This gastric band procedure, also known as VBG, involves the same band used during the sleeve gastrectomy, which is placed around the stomach. The stomach is then stapled above the band to form a small pouch, which in some sense shrinks the stomach to produce the same effects. The procedure has been noted as a successful one to lose weight compared to many other types of weight-loss surgeries. Even though compared to the sleeve gastrectomy, it may seem like a less complicated surgery, it has a higher complication rate. That is why it is considered far less common. Until today, there are only 5% of bariatric surgeons perform this particular gastric band surgery. Nevertheless, it is known for producing results and can still be used in hypnotherapy to produce similar results without the complications.

- Mixed Surgery (Restrictive and Malabsorptive) - This type of gastric band surgery forms a crucial part of most types of weight loss surgeries. It is more commonly referred to as gastric bypass and is done first, prior to other weight-loss surgeries. It also involves stapling the stomach and creates a shape of an intestine down the line of your stomach. This is done to ensure the patient consumes less food, referred to as restrictive mixed surgery, combined with malabsorptive surgery, meaning to absorb less food in the body.

What you need to know about hypnotic gastric band therapy

If you're wondering whether gastric band surgery is right for you, you may want to consider getting the hypnotherapy version thereof.

Hypnotherapy is the perfect alternative, is 100% safe as opposed to surgery which has many complications, and also a lot more affordable. It has a success rate of more than 90% in patients, which is why more people prefer it over gastric band surgery. Given that you can also conduct it in the comfort of your own home, you don't even have to worry about the cost involved. Overall it serves as a very convenient way to slim down, essentially shrinking your stomach.

Again, hypnosis doesn't involve any physical procedure involving surgery. It is a safe alternative that uses innovative and developed technology to help you get where you want to be. The hypnotherapy session involves visualizing a virtual gastric band being fitted around your stomach that allows you to have the same experience as you initially would during surgery, but without the discomfort, excessive costs and inconvenience.

The effect is feeling as if you are hungry for longer periods, require less food, and experiencing a feeling of being full, even if you've only eaten half of your regular-sized portion. This will also help you make healthier choices and discover that you can indeed develop a much healthier relationship with food then you currently have.

If you're wondering whether gastric band hypnotherapy will work for you,

you have to ask yourself whether you have the imagination to support your session. Now, of course, everybody has an imagination, but is yours reasonable enough?

If you can close your eyes and imagine yourself looking at something in front of you that is not there, and spend time focusing on it, then you can make it through gastric band hypnotherapy successfully.

It's normal to think before you start anything, that if it isn't tailored to you specifically, it is likely to fail. However, visual gastric band hypnosis can offer you emotional healing. This supports your goals, including weight loss and health restoration. If you spend time engaging in it, you will learn that you can achieve whatever you set your intention on. You can remove your cravings subconsciously, eliminate any negative and emotional stress, as well as memories that form a part of your emotional eating pattern. Given that emotionality forms a big part of weight gain, you should know that it can be removed from your conscious mind through hypnotherapy and serve any individual willing to try it.

Gastric band hypnotherapy has a 95% success rate among patients, according to a clinical study conducted in the U.K. This study also proved that most people will be able to accept and succeed in hypnotherapy, but if they're not open to the experience, they won't find it helpful at all. People who are too closed off from new ideas, like hypnotherapy, which is often made out to be a negative practice among the uneducated, won't be able to relax properly for a hypnotherapist's words to take effect. (Engle, 2019)

After just one hypnotherapy session, you will know if it works, as it is supposed to start working after just one session. That is why hypnotherapy is not recommended for everyone. It's only suggested to anyone ready to change their feelings toward food. If you don't believe in it or that it will get you to where you want to go on your weight loss journey, it is deemed useless.

The cost of gastric band hypnotherapy sessions with a professional hypnotherapist can only be established after you've undergone an evaluation. Usually, every new patient requires up to five sessions in person. During these sessions, energy therapy techniques are also taught, which will help assist any struggle a patient may have with anxiety, anger, stress, and any other negative emotion.

Chapter 6:

The Gold Protocol:

The 21-day hypnotic method with daily affirmations

This guided weight loss meditation session is designed for you to reach your weight loss goals and lasts for 21 days. During this period, you will not only create a new habit that will support a sense of positivity and your mental well-being, but you will also experience achieving a sense of fulfillment as you set out to reach your goals.

Perhaps one of the biggest takeaways from guided hypnotherapy is learning that you are, in fact, in control of your own habits and that you can alter it as you please.

It is something that no one can take away from you or demotivate you for as you experience it in silence, on your own, and within your unconscious mind. Although it may sound like an incredible challenge to open yourself up to a 21-day persistent and daily hypnosis challenge, you should remind yourself that you are improving your life with each day performing this session. It's not only recommended for weight loss but also aids in your mental and emotional well-being. While you focus on practicing mindfulness and altering eating habits, you will also find that your mind shifts to a point where you are comfortable consciously implementing the same way of thinking in other areas of your life. This in return, presents a lot of positive energy in your life and allows you to focus on what you can control. This also eliminates stress, anxiety, depression, and allows you to become in tune with yourself more than ever before.

The gold protocol: A 21-Day hypnotic method for weight loss

Welcome to the gold protocol, a 21-day hypnotic method for weight loss.

The brain is a mechanism that can continue to change in our lifetime. The more you listen to this recording, the deeper the new habits and beliefs will go.

Know that it is never too late for positive change. Please never listen to this recording while driving, operating any type of machinery, while taking care of others, or any other duties. Please find a time when you can give this 100% your attention, preferably sitting down in a quiet space where you will not be interrupted.

When you're ready, please get yourself comfortable, settling in while sitting down.

As you sit, just start to slow down. Making time seems to be the hardest part, so just relax in knowing that the hardest part is now over. As you relax and settle in, just know that any movement, any adjustment or anything you need to do to become even more comfortable, will only aid in your relaxation. Feel free to move and adjust as needed.

As you relax, feeling your body, neck, and head completely supported, start to connect to your breathing. Feel your chest rise and fall while slowing down. Place all your focus for the next few seconds on your breathing, breathing in and out slowly. Breathe in calm and breathing out any thoughts or tension and stress, letting go with every breath. Send a wave of relaxation down your entire body and mind. With every breath, let go and sink into the floor or chair you are sitting in. Breathing out your negative thoughts, focus on sending them away to a different place that you are not focused on.

Follow your breath, knowing that anything truly important will come back at the right time. Breathing in space into the mind, clearing up empty thoughts with every exhale.

Letting go of thoughts, of any tension and extra energy in the mind.

Slowing down.

Finding your own pace.

As you breathe, feel your body rise and fall, with the gentle inhale and exhale of thoughts. Just trust yourself to let go.

With the next breath, focus on sending this breath up and into the face. Feel it melting every muscle in the cheeks, up to the eyes, feeling relaxation flow through your entire face, loosening and relaxing any tension. Send this all the way up into your forehead, smoothing out any tightness.

With the next breath now, send it up and over the top of the head, relaxing all the muscles surrounding the skull, feeling the back of your head, and the contact points of the floor or your chair. Just feeling your head relax, sinking back deeper and deeper. Now send this breath of relaxation down and around your neck, lengthening and loosening the neck, breathing freely. Open up the airways, and feel all the muscles in your neck letting go, relaxing and lengthening, feeling it ripple all the way to the shoulder blades and down. Feeling your shoulder blades sinking deeper into your chair or your upright posture.

Now send a wave of relaxation to your core, down your stomach and deep into your hips. Send it down into your seat while sinking down. Send the breath all the way down into the fingertips, through the elbows, flowing down into the wrists and hands, filling up completely with calm and relaxation. Exhale any resistance, accepting only calm, and send the next breath now down into your legs. Send into your thighs and knees, into your calves, and even down into your feet to the very tips of your toes. Let go more and more with every breath, melting every muscle, and as your breathing gets easier and easier as your rest into this space. Imagine now that your relaxation will deepen as I count you down into deeper levels, starting from 10 to 1.

10 - Feel your muscles just melt away, sinking down now.

9 - Becoming more and more relaxed, staying connected to your breath.

8 - Letting go of any last thoughts, dissolving them, trusting this process.

7 - Coming back to the breath, staying with the breath.

6 - Deep, deep down.

5 - Halfway down now, doubling your state of calm.

4 - With your whole body giving in, allowing gravity to support you from the top of your head to the tips of your toes.

3 - Your whole body is getting heavier and heavier, your eyelids are relaxed.

2 - Face relaxed, jaw loose.

1 - Coming to rest, feeling the mind open up in this quiet, safe space that is designated just for you.

As you feel the outside world fade away into the background, hearing all outside sounds and inside sounds blend together, like distant ocean waves, just becoming more connected to your inner self, your body sensations, your mind and emotions. Know that you are ready to begin your journey, and knowing that your mind is always alert, knowing that it will draw attention to anything urgent in your environment. You can let go, let go completely, and focus on the feeling in your body, and the sound of my voice. Knowing that everything you need to achieve your goals lies within you. Notice how you can feel a connection in your breath, down into your lungs, becoming more and more aware of your mind and your body.

Notice how so often we are unaware of the body. We separate the body, from the neck up, and treat almost everything as a stranger from the neck down.

Now is the time to re-engage, to live as a whole, from the top of your head to the tips of your toes and everything between. Becoming aware of your breathing and your heartbeat, and building on this mind-body connection, you are becoming more and more in-tuned of how shallow or deep your breathing is. Of the speed or slowness of your heartbeat, and the level of fullness or true hunger of your stomach.

Notice the feelings in your stomach. Notice the nerve-endings around your stomach. Can you feel them?

Perhaps your stomach awareness is just starting or getting stronger and will only strengthen. Start to become aware, feeling your level of appetite or fullness, and imagine now a scale of 1 to 10, or maybe a dial tone that turns up as you eat. See the numbers clearly labeled from 1 to 10, with one being unbearably starving, unable to think about anything other than food, and 10 being stuffed, unbearably full, sluggish, and slow to move.

See the numbers or the scale. Zoom in on each of these numbers, and wherever you feel this scale, whether around your stomach or in your mind's eye, make this as real and vivid as possible. Perhaps the numbers are red at each end of the scale, when you are starving or overly-stuffed. Between the extremes, of 1 starving and 10 stuffed, is the healthy zone between 3 and 7 with 3 or 4 where your body calls attention, with the need to eat. A pleasant emptiness, an anticipation of filling up with nutrition or a greater enjoyment of food. When you get to the number 7, imagine feeling entirely satisfied, three-quarters full, still with energy to move, feeling refueled, and ready to get on with your day. Focusing on an ideal zone between a 3 and a 7, never letting your hunger dip below a 3,

never letting your satisfaction going beyond a 7 to stuffed.

In the same way that you can and are retraining your brain, with repeated listening you are strengthening your neural networks, the wiring between your brain and stomach. If at any time you are unsure, you may pause again for a few moments and serve yourself a cool, refreshing glass of water to differentiate between thirst and true appetite. If you ever reach a level 3 or 4, you will be aware that it is time to eat, observing your regular natural rhythm of eating, and if it is a 5 or above, it is a sign that you need something else to satisfy you. Perhaps physical activity to burn off nervous tension or perhaps a conversation or kind word from a friend. Perhaps something to fill up your mind, and you will find it easier and easier to distinguish appetite from other needs, other types of hunger. This includes emotional hunger, mental hunger or physical hunger, and imagine yourself now at home back in the kitchen.

Visualize this scene, notice the colors of the cupboards, the fridge, the oven. Feel yourself there, and watch yourself getting ready for a meal, taking a few extra seconds before your mealtime. Take a few deep breaths in and out to become calm and present before every meal. As you get ready to eat, enjoy your gentle appetite. Feel it to slowly build, knowing that with an appetite, you will enjoy each mouthful even more. Starting out with a few extra seconds, a few seconds to put food on a plate or a bowl, and to find a seat because putting food on a plate or in a bowl assures that it enters your conscious awareness. No more distracted or semi-conscious eating, full awareness eating only. In the simple act of preparing food, giving yourself a place to sit comfortably is an act of self-respect, treating yourself as you would a guest. As you look at the food on a plate or bowl, you'll have a few more seconds to take in a smell, the look of the meal you are about to enjoy, treating yourself as one of your best guests.

As you visualize yourself in your kitchen and home, preparing food, connecting to your appetite, diffusing from any emotions related to your true appetite, you realize that you deserve to experience every mouthful. That whatever you are putting in your body, you deserve the taste, the texture. As much as life can be busy, you turn mealtimes into priorities. Over the next few days, those next few seconds you give to focus will expand into minutes, and with every meal, you will slow down to a point where you spend at least 20 minutes on every meal. You will start learning that the brain needs at least 20-minute signals from the stomach, between the moment that it is pleasantly satisfied and energized. Dial-up your

internal signals while dialing down on external signals and distractions. Relaxing, and sitting down for every bite, every meal, every snack.

You know that you need to feel enjoyment from food, as well as nutrition from food, and for that reason, you tune out all the unnecessary distractions surrounding you. As you deserve to taste everything that you eat, you're going to start to take smaller, more mindful mouthfuls. Smaller mouth-fulls, ensuring that every bite you taste, slowly rolls over your tongue. Every texture is felt between your teeth. With the first mouthful, your stomach nerves start to engage and pick up the signals as your stomach slowly starts to fill. Feeling the electricity run from your stomach to your brain, those long nerve-endings engaging, monitoring this mealtime. Between every bite, you will take on the simple habit of placing down your fork or spoon if hand-held. You will now get into a regular rhythm of eating, eating a bite and putting everything down.

As you focus on what you are eating, enjoying it right now. As you swallow picking up the food, taking another bite and then put it down, shifting away from what is remaining on your plate to what you are eating at this moment. Acknowledge the feeling of your appetite going slowly up. As you learn to engage in a regular rhythm of mouthfuls, so too will you engage in a regular rhythm of mealtimes. Building solid habits of mindful eating, building and maintaining your ideal weight.

Whenever you get to a level 6 or 7, feel your stomach reach a level of 3 or 4 quarters full. Just see yourself pushing the bowl or plate away from you, getting up and leaving, feeling enough energy getting up and away, allowing yourself to get on with your day and getting rid of any food on your plate. It may be in the garbage, compost, or wrapped up for later. You are now no longer driven by external signals. There will always be more food. You have a lifetime of access to food. What matters is enjoyment and nutrition, and once you get to a level 7, you are no longer enjoying your food. You have received all the nutrition you need and are no longer enjoying your meal. Also, treat yourself with respect to now longer use yourself as a garbage can. As you rediscover the act of conscious eating, easing into this, adding just a few more seconds to every mealtime, perhaps only now you are starting to believe that focusing on what you eat is only important after you learn how to eat and why you eat.

As you dial into your internal signals, you dial into all the external signals, whether peer or family pressure, advertising, or the latest fad, you realize that long-term change happens slowly.

Allowing the mind to ease into new habits, knowing that the mind rejects certain changes, as you may have found with certain diets and strict regimes. With repeated listening, building new pathways in your brand. With repeated listening, building new habits for a lifetime. It is the greatest feeling to know that thinking yourself slim lies in such simple, yet effective principles.

Know that the number one rule of slim people doesn't involve any special diet. It is simply connecting to their appetite and slowing down. That's right. Slowing down and enjoying every bite, meal, or snack.

In a moment now, I'm going to count you out from 1 to 10, and on 10, you will open your eyes, coming back to the present time in this present place.

Before I do so, just congratulate yourself for the good work you have done today.

1 - Stay connected with the body and mind, feeling the signals get stronger and stronger between the stomach and brain.

2 - Notice how much calmer and more relaxed you are than just a few minutes ago.

3 - Remind yourself that you are so much stronger when you tune into your body's wisdom and natural signals.

4 - Remember to slow down every time you go to eat, taking three deep breaths in and out.

5 - Commit to gauging your appetite, confirm that you are at a level 3 or 4. Drink a tall glass of water and differentiate between thirst and appetite.

6 - Come up higher, feeling energy circulate.

7 - Feel so good from head to toe.

8 - Know that you will only eat to a level of satisfaction–to a level 6 or 7.

9 - Remember to channel any false appetite, any emotional, physical or mental energy in the right way in a 10-minute boost of activity or connection with yourself.

10 - Come back up, eyes open, wide awake.

Just notice now how relaxed and energized you are, staying with your mind-body connection.

Following this 21-day gold protocol hypnosis for weight loss challenge, you will create the building blocks for a successful weight loss journey to attain and maintain your ideal healthy weight.

Mindful affirmations to live by

- I am committed to my health and healing.
- I feel better in my skin.
- I feel energized and content.
- Good health is my nature.
- Abundant health is my birthright.
- It feels great to be in shape.
- I eat less and move more.
- I make consistent, healthy choices.
- I love the wide variety of healthy food choices I have.
- I am creative with my meal planning and enjoy cooking.
- I am a responsible, conscious eater.
- I love life and the rich potential it holds.
- My mind and body are wired for success.
- I love and accept myself fully.
- I am committed to my health and longevity.
- I do this for myself, and all the people I love.
- I serve as a positive example for others.
- I have many gifts to share with the world.

- The world needs my talents and appreciate my perspective.
- Good health allows me to share my gifts and leave a legacy.
- I create my future with the decisions I make right now.
- I let go of health choices that don't serve me.
- I let go of guilt and shame.
- I let go of sadness and depression.
- I embrace this new, bright era of my life.
- I believe in myself and in my ability to thrive.
- I give myself permission to feel good.
- I respect and care for my body.
- Healthy living is my way of life.
- I respect and care for my body.
- Healthy living is a long-term, and a sustainable habit.
- Healthy living is my way of life, and I prefer it compared to unhealthy living.
- I love my healthy lifestyle.
- I am fully committed to feeling better.
- I am healthy and whole.

Chapter 7:

Tips and Tricks

To achieve your weight loss goals, you must be willing to let any fear and doubt you may have about hypnotherapy, go. It is not something that you can second guess, particularly not its effectivity and results-driven orientation. It is a solution used for many different reasons, even other than weight loss. Hypnotherapy for weight loss can help you overcome a negative relationship with food, one that may have formed over a period or throughout your entire life. It is something that can present you with proper results and that you can always be certain of.

Although it is not a diet or weight loss supplement, it fulfills a similar supporting role and serves as the foundation on the journey of living a more mindful lifestyle. Since the method thereof is focused on replacing old negative habits with new positive ones, it really helps one to overcome challenges faced when trying to lose weight.

Whether you want to opt for a one-on-one weight loss for hypnotherapy session or just listen to audiobooks online, both can serve you usefully.

Before you dive into the world of hypnotherapy, you should know that there's a lot more to it than you may have initially thought. Much like Yoga and meditation, in general, it serves a greater purpose as it leads you on to a mindful path of physical, mental, and emotional wellness.

Tips for hypnosis for weight loss

- Find the right hypnotherapist for weight loss for you. How would you go about doing this, you may ask? Instead of going the obvious route of searching for hypnotherapists online in your area, why not ask for recommendations instead? Honestly, what's better than asking a friend, family member, or acquaintance to recommend you a good hypnotherapist for weight loss? If no one you know, knows a hypnotherapist that is known for the outstanding jobs they perform, then you may want to check with your doctor and ask for advice. They should be able to recommend a qualified and results-oriented hypnotherapist for weight loss. To ensure you have the right hypnotherapist once you've found one, be sure to check with yourself whether their consultation felt as though it was thorough, whether the hypnotherapy program was adjusted to meet your needs if there were any, and whether the practitioner was helpful and answered all of your questions. When hypnotherapists allow for space between sessions, it's also an indication that you're dealing with a good hypnotherapist.

- Don't pay any attention to advertising. We live in 2019, which means that everything we see online is taken seriously. However, it shouldn't be. People are oblivious and susceptible to accept everything they read or hear, but when it comes to advertising, not everything can be trusted. Advertising should, ever so often, be disregarded and not taken too seriously as it can be very misleading. It's always better to conduct your own research before you simply accept that something is a certain way or not. In the case of hypnotherapy, since there are so many negative associations related to the practice, it's best to find out what's it all about yourself. As you can see from this useful set of information provided about hypnotherapy for weight loss, it is completely safe and probably nothing negative that you expected it to be.

- Get information about training, qualifications, and necessary experience. Before you pick a hypnotherapist, you must be sure about their basic information first. Do they run their own practice or operate independently? Are they certified and have a license? Ensuring that they also adhere to ethical standards, most preferably recommended by other medical physicians, you'll be assured that you are dealing with someone who knows what they are doing.

- Before choosing one hypnotherapist, talk to several first. Perhaps one of the best ways to find out whether a hypnotherapist is best suited for you is to talk with a few of them over a phone call first. This will take some effort, but it will be worth it in the end. You have to consider whether they can relate to you, care about your well-being and listen to your concerns, whether they are personable, accommodating, and professional. If they tick all the boxes, then you're good to go.

- Don't fall for any promises that may sound unrealistic. If a hypnotist tells you that their therapy session will help you lose weight fast, then don't even bother going to a single session. In reality, hypnosis for weight loss is a process that takes time. It can take anywhere between three weeks, up to three months to see your physical body change and to lose weight. Since your body and mind should first adjust, you need to allow time for it to do so. Hypnosis for weight loss isn't a fad, nor is it a means of losing weight overnight. It's also important to avoid hypnotherapists who suggest they will make you lose weight. Since they will only be talking during the session what they're telling you is not true whatsoever. What you can expect from a professional and authentic hypnotherapist, however, is a professional individual who takes responsibility for helping you to get where you want to go. This person should help you access your subconscious mind with ease, and help you bring it on board with a proper weight loss plan and possibly an exercise routine.

- Is your hypnotherapist of choice multi-skilled? Even though hypnosis is a terrific tool and can alter the mind's way of thinking about food, it goes hand-in-hand with nutrition. This is something you need to consider, especially whether your hypnotist has a good understanding of what it takes for you to lose weight sustainably and healthily. Many people focused on starting a weight loss journey don't necessarily know what they should do or what they should eat. When looking for a hypnotherapist, look for one that has a self-help coaching or some type of psychotherapy qualification, as well as a qualification/background in either nutrition or cognitive behavioral therapy.

- Find out the time you should engage in a program. This is quite important as hypnotherapy can become quite expensive if you're going to a professional for one-on-one sessions. If you prefer going to a professional rather than conducting the sessions at your home, you can choose to spread your sessions out over time to make it more affordable. Even though you may think that the sessions become less effective to achieve the overall effect, it works more effectively as your mind and body requires time to adjust. Time is also required as you change your old habits and replace them with new ones to lose weight.

- Ask your hypnotherapist if they can provide you with a program to maintain your progress at home. A recording particularly helps to allow you to spread out sessions over time. Listening to your weight loss hypnosis recording every day will keep you in check and help you stay motivated and focused.

- As your hypnotherapist if they can tailor-make your hypnotherapy weight loss program for you. If they agree to it, you can expect a weight loss hypnotherapy program that is much more effective than individualized hypnosis, offering treatments that may work better than ones that cater to everyone. Since every person is different compared to others, this makes a lot more sense. Sure, the general program will work, but a personalized one could offer you better results.

- Ask whether your program includes an introduction session. Starting with hypnotherapy for weight loss, you don't want to just dive right into it. It's important to take the necessary time, even if it's just an hour, to establish your needs and concerns regarding your current habits, lifestyle, and goals with your hypnotherapist. Ensuring that they care about your well-being and results instead of just taking you through the session is equally important. Taking the time to talk to your hypnotherapist and getting to know them better will help you feel more at ease and form a foundation of trust before starting with your hypnotherapy sessions.

- Establish the costs involved before starting with your sessions. Ensuring you know how much an initial consultation and each session costs will be another important factor you have to consider before choosing a hypnotherapist. Considering the cost, consider an overview of their program compared to other potential weight loss programs, review the cost solely based on the quality of service you'll receive, and take into account that you can spread your program over weeks instead of going to a few sessions a week.

Lastly, you should view hypnotherapy as an investment in yourself and well-being, rather than an unnecessary expense. The context for this thought will realize once you engage in, or completed your program.

Conclusion

Hypnosis is used for many different reasons today, something that once was thought of as a magic trick or something that doesn't work. However, looking at results curated by clients over the years, especially with weight loss, one can see that it is indeed something that can help you to get ahead in life. Apart from losing weight, it can help you overcome your fears, stress, anxiety, depression, and even support your mental well-being when faced with addiction, sleep deprivation, challenges, and more.

It also contributes as a major factor supporting health and wellness, allowing you to practice mindfulness, which is something many individuals don't know how to do. It aids as a psychological treatment that can help you experience far more benefits to serve your well-being than you ever thought was possible. It allows you to experience changes in your thoughts, behaviors, perceptions and sensations, and can be performed in either a clinical setting or the comfort of your own home.

Hypnosis has successfully proven to improve deep sleep in individuals by up to 80%, which allows one to wake up more energized and refreshed each day. Since sleep plays such a vital role in our everyday lives and is needed to sustain

our health, it just goes to show how beneficial hypnosis can actually be.

After experiencing this audiobook, you are most certainly aware of the incredible benefits that hypnosis for weight loss holds in store for you.

To refresh your mind about the benefits you could experience by following one of our hypnosis for weight loss sessions, our listed wellness benefits include:

- It helps to rectify sleep patterns, such as insomnia, sleepwalking, and having general trouble sleeping. If you suffer from any of these issues, you can learn how to relax your brain and form better sleeping patterns by following a hypnotherapy program daily. Given that hypnotherapy aids in fixing any issues related to improper sleep, it also serves your weight loss journey, as sleep is required to maintain a proper-functioning body and mind. It also assists your metabolism in operating correctly, which helps you lose weight, restores the cells in your body, and ensures the proper harmonious functioning of your entire body.

- It helps to reduce anxiety and depression. Since anxiety and depression are experienced due to an imbalance of emotions and being overly affected by the daily stresses of life, hypnotherapy works by relaxing the mind, allowing patients to become in town with themselves and attain a sense of control and mindfulness in their lives. Hypnotherapy is tailored to allow you to let go of any negative thoughts, habits, and daily experiences you may have, shifting your focus on positive things. Given that a lot of health issues stem from anxiety, including irregular breathing, high blood pressure, heart diseases, and has the potential to create an overall imbalance in the body, hypnotherapy serves as the perfect option to control any stress or anxiety you may experience. As stress and anxiety are the biggest contributors to overeating, lack of portion control, and emotional eating, it's yet another reason why it can aid in significant weight loss. Since hypnotherapy is focused on fixing the mind, everything else usually aligns perfectly.

- It helps to reduce the symptoms associated with irritable bowel syndrome symptoms (IBS). Hypnotherapy can completely relieve symptoms associated with IBS, including constipation, bloating, and diarrhea. It can also improve bowel movements and support a balanced metabolism, which prevents secondary disruptive symptoms, like fatigue, nausea, backache, and urinary tract issues.

- It helps you to quit addictions. Since most people turn toward addiction to help get rid of their problems as a result of stress, anxiety, depression or emotional issues, it's simple to understand why hypnotherapy can help one quit bad habits, including smoking, alcoholism, an addiction to medication or pain killers, and most relevantly, an addiction to food. Hypnotherapy allows you to train your mind to take whatever your addiction is and form a type of resistance toward it in your subconscious, which eventually translates into your conscious thinking.

- It helps to reduce chronic pain and symptoms associated with feeling unwell. Hypnotherapy's purpose is to not only help you overcome a lot of obstacles in your life but also to make you feel like you are on top of the world. It serves as a great method to help you overcome symptoms associated with illness or stress in your body and can take your overall wellness to a whole new level.

Taking chemotherapy for cancer patients as an example, even though patients often want to give up, they shouldn't. Since the mind can determine whether we are sick or not, hypnotherapy can help alter the mind and make one believe that they are getting healthier. With this positive incentive placed in the mind, patients will only focus on getting better and not on the severity of their diagnosis. Hypnotherapy can indeed help cancer patients stay positive, and thus speed up their recovery, serving even an even greater purpose as those who lack positivity during chemotherapy are more likely to give up early and pass.

- It can help you lose weight!

After reviewing the endless benefits hypnotherapy presents you with, we can conclude that it is indeed a practice of divine intention and medicine, blissfully combined to create the best version of yourself than you ever thought was possible. Whether you're suffering from obesity, you're a little overweight, you suffer from health issues that contribute to your struggle in not losing weight...

It doesn't matter what your reason is as to why you can't lose weight. There is always a reason why you can turn your can't into a can.

In truth, losing weight is not rocket science. It is quite simple and can be achieved, no matter where you're at in your life or how difficult you may think you have it. Focusing on weight loss, we have also established the importance of focusing on the overall recovery of your body, which serves you every day.

It demands respect and will serve you even better if you can manage to resist the temptations life throws at you ever so often, and in some cases every day. Learning principles in nutrition, such as the fact that sugar is a killer and that white-based flour carbohydrates are not your friend, can serve as a massive asset in your journey toward achieving wellness, among many other things.

To make your journey easier, it's also a much better idea to focus on wellness instead of a number on the scale. Weight loss will occur if your intentions are set right. You know who you are as a person, and so, you can either remain the same or choose to grow. Since your mind is connected to your body, and the two require each other to survive, you must ensure that both operate harmoniously together. Only then, will you see results, survive this incredible journey, and attain success in all you wish to achieve.

Reaching the end of this audiobook and concluding with the many benefits hypnotherapy can present you with, you should be aware that your body is your home. It is a place that you identify with as safe and complete in your very own way. Without your body, you can't do anything, and so, to do everything, you must ensure it is sustained going into the future.

References

WebMD, (n.d.), Hypnotherapy - Hypnosis

Retrieved from URL

https://www.webmd.com/mental-health/mental-health-hypnotherapy#1

Bauer, B. A, 2018, Is weight-loss hypnosis effective?

Retrieved from URL

https://www.mayoclinic.org/healthy-lifestyle/weight-loss/expert-answers/weight-loss-hypnosis/faq-20058291

Zimberoff, D. (2018), What is the difference between hypnosis and hypnotherapy? How does hypnotherapy work?

Retrieved from URL

https://web.wellness-institute.org/blog/bid/256330/what-is-the-difference-between-hypnosis-and-hypnotherapy

Lefave, S. (2019) What is hypnosis for weight loss -And does it work?

Retrieved from URL

https://www.oprahmag.com/life/health/a28187126/hypnosis-for-weight-loss/

Anderson, C. H. (n.d.), Everything you need to know about hypnosis for weight loss

Retrieved from URL

https://www.shape.com/weight-loss/tips-plans/everything-you-need-know-about-hypnosis-weight-loss

Your Tango, (n.d.), If your struggle to lose weight, there's a new way to help shed those stubborn pounds

Retrieved from URL

https://www.yourtango.com/experts/DeniAbbie/how-lose-weight-loss-hypnosis-why-works

Ledochowski, I. (2019), Hypnosis for weight loss: A complete guide to the 5 key reasons people gain weight & the techniques you can use to overcome them

Retrieved from URL

https://hypnosistrainingacademy.com/using-hypnosis-for-weight-loss/

Weiss, S. (2017), I tried hypnosis to change my terrible eating habits

Retrieved from URL

https://www.self.com/story/hypnosis-healthy-eating-habits

Marie Claire, (2015), Think yourself thin: 7 secrets behind hypnosis for weight loss

Retrieved from URL

https://www.marieclaire.co.uk/life/health-fitness/think-yourself-thin-7-secrets-behind-hypnosis-for-weightloss-74656

Resultan, J. (n.d.), How to self-hypnotize for weight loss

Retrieved from URL

https://www.livestrong.com/article/345781-how-to-self-hypnotize-for-weight-loss/

City/Hypnosis blog, (n.d.), The top 10 reasons to use weight loss hypnotherapy

Retrieved from URL

https://www.cityhypnosis.com/blog/weight-loss-hypnotherapy/

Meridian Peak Hypnosis, (n.d.),

Retrieved from URL

https://www.meridianpeakhypnosis.com/portion-control-lose-weight/

Uncommon knowledge, (n.d.), Regain portion control and start eating the right amount

Retrieved from URL

https://www.hypnosisdownloads.com/weight-loss/portion-control

Roger, (2013), Overcoming portion control and overeating

Retrieved from URL

https://hypnosishealthinfo.com/portion-control-overeating/

Hypnosis for Weight Loss: Using Hypnotherapy to Shed Pounds, (n.d.),

Retrieved from URL

https://gshypnosis.com/hypnosis-for-weight-loss-using-hypnotherapy-to-shed-pounds-2/

Hypnotherapy Directory, (n.d.), Gastric band hypnotherapy

https://www.hypnotherapy-directory.org.uk/articles/gastric-band.html

MacGill, M, (2018), How does a gastric band work?

Retrieved from URL

https://www.medicalnewstoday.com/articles/298313.php#other_options

Engle, B. (2019), 6 Things you should know about gastric band hypnotherapy

Retrieved from URL

https://www.englehypnotherapy.com/blog/gastric-band-hypnosis/

WebMD, (n.d.), What is gastric banding surgery for weight loss

Retrieved from URL

https://www.webmd.com/diet/obesity/gastric-banding-surgery-for-weight-loss#1

Sweeney, S. (n.d.), Weight loss hypnotists - 11 Tips for finding the best one for you

Retrieved from URL

https://www.onlinehypnotherapyclinic.com/weight-loss-hypnotists.html

Penn Medicine, (2019), 6 Surprising health benefits of hypnosis

Retrieved from URL

https://www.pennmedicine.org/updates/blogs/health-and-wellness/2019/january/hypnosis

THE EASY LECTIN FREE COOKBOOK

By

Lil Ron

Table of Contents

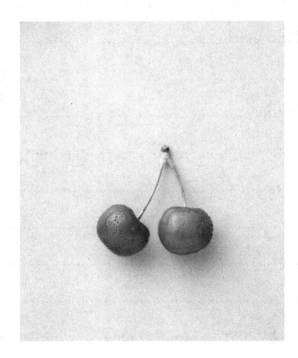

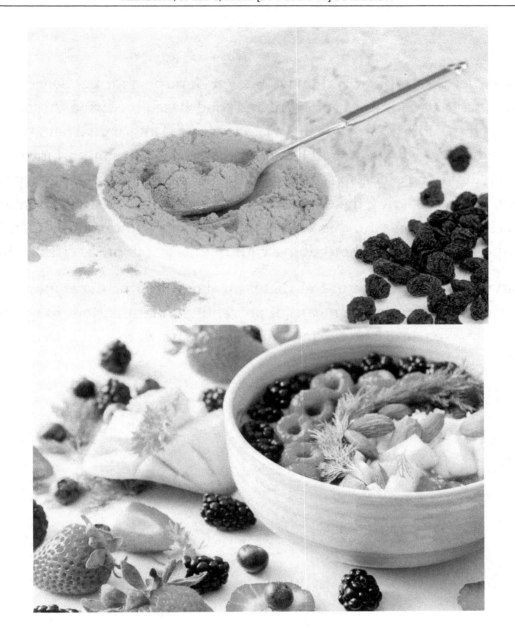

Introduction

The lectin-free diet was popularized by Dr. Steven Gundry, a former heart surgeon who has since switched his focus to supplement and food-based medicine. According to Gundry, removing lectins from your diet via a lectin-free alternative helps to reduce body weight while improving overall health in the process. It is important to note that the official version of the diet also requires that users purchase a proprietary supplement from Dr. Gundry so following the diet outlined in this book may not be as effective without it. With that being said, this book is **not** recommending going out and purchasing the supplement without doing your own research on its efficacy beforehand.

With that out of the way, the lectin-free diet is all about limiting the amount of lectin in the body to reasonable levels as a means of preventing inflammation from developing due to prolonged exposure. Chronic inflammation is known to lead to everything from arthritis, to cancer, to even death.

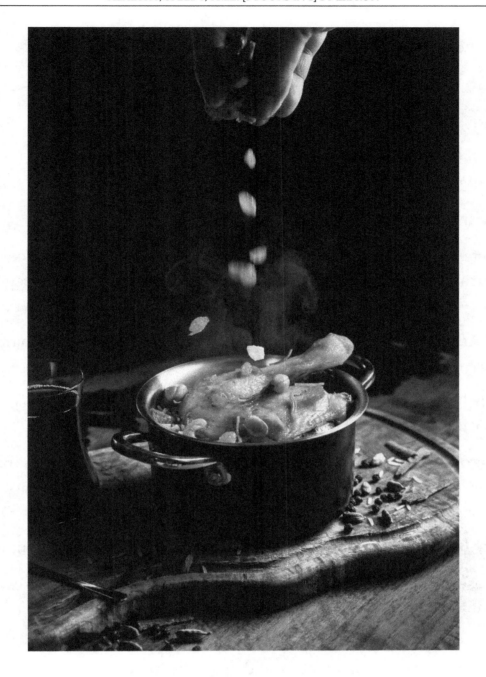

PART ONE:

The Lectin-Free Diet

How food affects your body

Uncontrolled inflammation, which may result from excessive Lectin input leads to a wide variety of different harmful side effects.

Some of them include:

Type 1 Diabetes: Type 1 Diabetes will cause the immune system to attack and destroy insulin-producing cells in your pancreas that will ultimately disrupt the regulation of sugar levels in your body.

Rheumatoid Arthritis: RA causes the immune system to attack specific joints that results in considerable discomfort and pain.

Psoriatic Arthritis: This causes the skin cell to multiply rapidly, which results in red and scaly patches called plaques on the skin.

Multiple Sclerosis: MS tends to damage the protective coating that surrounds nerve cells (known as myelin sheath) and affects the transmission of a neural message between the brain and body. This often leads to weakness, balance issues, etc.

Inflammatory Bowel Syndromes: This disease will irritate the intestinal lining.

Graves' Disease: This disease attacks the thyroid gland in your neck and causes it to produce too much hormone, which results in a severe imbalance.

Cancer: Cancerous tumors tend to secrete substances that attract cytokines and free-radicals that further cause inflammation and helps the tumors to survive. So, if you are already suffering from Anti-Inflammation, it will just make the condition of the Cancer much worse and help to grow and spread.

Alzheimer: The brain does not have any pain receptors, but that doesn't mean that it won't be able to feel the effects of inflammation. Researchers have recently discovered that people a high level of Omega-6 fatty acids tend to have a higher chance of suffering from Alzheimer's disease, which just put is a disease and hampers your memory and makes you keep forgetting things from time to time.

While there are a lot of benefits that you can reap from a Lectin Free diet in the long term, some of the more crucial ones are as follows:

1. You will lower the chances of suffering from chronic inflammation
2. You will improve your heart condition
3. It will protect you from cancer
4. It will help you fend off depression
5. It will help you to tackle various autoimmune diseases such as rheumatoid arthritis, diabetes and celiac diseases

Proofs that the lectin-free diet is useful

The lectin-free diet is all about limiting the amount of lectin in the body to reasonable levels as a means of preventing inflammation from developing due to prolonged exposure. Chronic inflammation is known to lead to everything from arthritis, to cancer, to even death.

According to the creator of the diet, Dr. Gundry, the following foods will ease you into the diet:

- Olives and Olive Oil: Olives are generally low in Lectin and are safe to consume on a Lectin free diet
- Avocados: Though it is a fruit, you can enjoy Avocados in Lectin free recipes
- Mushrooms: You can choose from a wide variety of mushrooms available in the market.
- Celery
- Asparagus
- Cruciferous Vegetables: veggies such as Brussels sprouts, broccoli, or cauliflower are veggies that provide you with great nutrients while being low in Lectins
- Sweet Potatoes: even if potatoes are considered to be high in Lectins, sweet potatoes are amazing for a Lectin Free diet. Enjoy the health benefits of potatoes while keeping your Lectins in check
- Pasture-raised meat: When considering meat, try to go for pasture-raised meat as they will help you meet up your daily protein need.

Lectin-free diet frequently asked questions

What are Lectins?

In the simplest terms, Lectins are the proteins that are responsible for binding cell membranes together.

They have a sugar binding nature and are the "Glyco" section of Glycoconjugates present on cell membranes.

They help to assist other cells to interact with each other and joint together without the help of the immune mechanism. Lectins are considered to be a key factor when considering inter-cell bindings.

Why Are Lectins Bad for Us?

While Lectin is found in almost all parts of the plants, the "Seeds" are the ones that humans tend to consume the most and are considered to be one of the original ways through which humans are exposed to Lectins.

According to various recent studies, it has been found that Lectins are incredibly toxic to the human body.

These harmful proteins tend to cause widespread inflammation all around the body, which leads to severe various side effects including, but not limited to unwanted weight gain, fogginess, and digestion issues and so on.

All these side-effects have given Lectins the notorious title of being "Anti-Nutrients" as they not only cause inflammation but also restrict the absorption of essential nutrients required by the body.

What are Glutens?

Before the discovery of Lectins, Glutens were perhaps one of the most controversial entities that often force people into debates of whether it was good or bad.

There is a powerful connection between Glutens and Lectins! But before establishing and explaining that, I do believe that it is essential for you to have an understanding of what "Glutens" actually are.

Strictly speaking, Glutens are a family of protein found in grains such as barley, wheat, rye, and spelled!

Perhaps the most common Gluten contain grain that we mostly consume is Wheat.

When flour is mixed up with water, Gluten is responsible for the texture that you get. This glue-like property helps the dough to be elastic and allows bread to rise when baked.

However, it seems that there is a large chunk of the population who are unable to tolerate gluten.

While most people can digest it just fine, others tend to suffer from various diseases such as wheat allergy, inflammation, irritable bowel syndrome, celiac diseases and so on.

What is Inflammation?

And this brings us to our next issue with Lectins and Glutens, Inflammation.

It seems that amongst the many side effects of Lectins exposure, Inflammation stands at the top of the list! But what does inflammation mean?

Let me elaborate

Inflammation is a vital aspect of our body's immune system and is an attempt to heal itself from any anomaly/defend itself from foreign organisms such as bacteria, virus and of course, repair damaged tissues.

Without natural inflammation, the wound's in our body would never heal and infections would eventually become deadly!

PART TWO:

Lectin-Free Recipes

Breakfast recipes

Mesmerizing Cauliflower Pudding

Servings: 4

Prep +cook time: 20 minutes

Ingredients

- 1 and ½ cups unsweetened coconut milk
- 1 cup water
- 1 cup cauliflower rice (florets pulsed in food processor)
- 2 teaspoon organic ground cinnamon powder
- 1 teaspoon pure vanilla extract
- Pinch of salt

Directions

1. Add the listed ingredients to your Instant Pot and stir
2. Lock lid and cook on HIGH pressure for 20 minutes
3. Release pressure naturally over 10 minutes. Serve and enjoy!

Cool Prosciutto Cane

Servings: 4

Prep +cook time: 7 minutes

Ingredients

- 1 pound thick asparagus
- 80 ounces prosciutto, sliced

Directions

1. Add the listed ingredients to your Instant Pot and stir
2. Lock lid and cook on HIGH pressure for 20 minutes
3. Release pressure naturally over 10 minutes. Serve and enjoy!

Creamy Nice Broccoli Casserole

Servings: 6

Prep +cook time: 6 hours 15 minutes

Ingredients

- 1 tablespoon extra-virgin olive oil
- 1 pound broccoli, cut into florets
- 1 pound cauliflower, cut into florets
- ¼ cup almond flour
- 2 cups coconut milk
- ½ teaspoon ground nutmeg
- Pinch of fresh ground black pepper
- 1 and ½ cups cashew cream

Directions

1. Grease the Slow Cooker inner pot with olive oil
2. Place broccoli and cauliflower to your Slow Cooker
3. Take a small bowl and stir in almond flour, coconut milk, pepper, 1 cup of cashew cream
4. Pour coconut milk mixture over vegetables and top casserole with remaining cashew cream
5. Cover and cook on LOW for 6 hours
6. Server and enjoy!

Bacon and Kale

Servings: 4

Prep +cook time: 6 hours 15 minutes

Ingredients

- 2 tablespoons bacon fat
- 2 pounds kale, rinsed and chopped
- 2 bacon slices, cooked and chopped
- 2 teaspoons garlic, minced
- 2 cups vegetable broth
- Salt as needed
- Fresh ground black pepper

Directions

1. Grease the inner pot with bacon fat
2. Add kale, garlic, bacon, broth to insert and toss. Cover and cook on LOW for 6 hours
3. Season with salt and pepper. Serve and enjoy!

Healthy Golden Mushrooms

Servings: 4

Prep +cook time: 6 hours 10 minutes

Ingredients

- 3 tablespoons extra virgin olive oil
- 1 pound button mushrooms, wiped, cleaned and halved
- 2 teaspoons garlic, minced
- ¼ teaspoon salt
- 1/8 teaspoon fresh ground black pepper
- 2 tablespoons fresh parsley, chopped

Directions

1. Add olive oil, mushrooms, garlic, salt, pepper to your Slow Cooker
2. Cover and cook on LOW for 6 hours
3. Serve toss with parsley. Enjoy!

Summer Vegetable Mélange

Servings: 4

Prep +cook time: 6 hours 15 minutes

Ingredients

- ½ cup extra virgin olive oil
- ¼ cup balsamic vinegar
- 1 tablespoon dried basil
- 1 teaspoon dried thyme
- ¼ teaspoon salt
- 2 cups cauliflower florets
- 1 yellow bell pepper, deseeded and cut into strips
- 1 cup button mushrooms, halved

Directions:

1. Take a large bowl and add oil, basil, vinegar, thyme, salt and whisk
2. Add cauliflower, bell pepper, mushrooms and toss well to coat
3. Transfer the veggies to Slow Cooker
4. Cover and cook on LOW for 6 hours
5. Serve and enjoy!

Cool Healthy Granola

Servings: 4

Prep +cook time: 4 hours 10 minutes

Ingredients

- ½ cup coconut oil
- 2 teaspoons vanilla extract
- 1 teaspoon maple extract
- 1 cup pecans, chopped
- 1 cup sunflower seeds
- 1 cup unsweetened shredded coconut
- ½ cup hazelnuts
- ½ cup slivered almonds
- 2 tablespoon stevia
- ½ teaspoon cinnamon
- ¼ teaspoon ground nutmeg
- ¼ teaspoon salt

Directions:

1. Grease the inner pot of your Slow Cooker with 1 tablespoon of coconut oil
2. Take a large bowl and add oil, vanilla and extract
3. Stir well and add pecans, coconut, sunflower seeds, hazelnuts, almonds, stevia, nutmeg, cinnamon and salt
4. Toss well
5. Transfer the mix to your Slow Cooker
6. Cover and cook on LOW for 3-4 hours
7. Transfer granola to baking sheet and cover with foil
8. Let it cool and serve as needed!

Tender Sweet Braised Cabbage

Servings: 6

Prep +cook time: 8 hours 10 minutes

Ingredients

- 1 tablespoon extra-virgin olive oil
- 1 small red cabbage, coarsely shredded
- ½ sweet onion, thinly sliced
- ¼ cup apple cider vinegar
- 3 tablespoon stevia
- 2 teaspoon garlic, minced
- ½ teaspoon ground nutmeg
- 1/8 teaspoon ground cloves
- 2 tablespoon ghee
- Salt as needed
- Fresh ground black pepper as needed
- ½ cup walnuts, chopped
- ½ cup cashew cream
- Peppercorns for garnish

Directions:

1. Grease the Slow Cooker with olive oil
2. Add cabbage, onion, vinegar, stevia, nutmeg, garlic, cloves to insert
3. Stir well
4. Add ghee all over the cabbage mix
5. Cover and cook on LOW for 7-8 hours
6. Season with salt and pepper
7. Serve with topping of walnuts, cashew cream and peppercorns
8. Enjoy!

Simple And Straightforward Broccoli

Servings: 2

Prep +cook time: 7 minutes

Ingredients

- 1 medium broccoli
- Salt and pepper as needed
- ¾ cup water

Directions:

1. Add ¾ cup of water to the pot
2. Chop up the broccoli into florets and place them on a steamer rack
3. Place the rack on top of your pot
4. Lock up the lid and cook on HIGH pressure for 2 minutes
5. Once done ,allow the pressure naturally
6. Serve with a seasoning of salt and pepper

Very Nutty Faux "Oatmeal"

Servings: 6

Prep +cook time: 8 hours 10 minutes

Ingredients:

- 1 tablespoon coconut oil
- 1 cup coconut milk
- 1 cup unsweetened shredded coconut
- ½ cup pecans, chopped
- ½ cup almonds, sliced
- 2 tablespoon stevia
- 1 avocado, diced
- 1 teaspoon ground cinnamon
- ¼ teaspoon ground nutmeg
- ½ cup blueberries, garnish

Directions:

1. Grease the inner pot of your Slow Cooker with coconut oil
2. Place coconut milk, coconut, pecans, almonds, avocado, stevia, cinnamon and nutmeg to your Slow Cooker
3. Cover and cook on LOW for 8 hours
4. Stir the mix until you have your desired texture
5. Serve topped with blueberries
6. Enjoy!

Early Morning Good Sausage Meatloaf

Servings: 6

Prep +cook time: 3 hours 10 minutes

Ingredients

- 1 tablespoon extra-virgin olive oil
- 2 pounds ground pork
- 1 sweet onion, chopped
- ½ cup almond flour
- 2 teaspoon garlic, minced
- 2 teaspoon dried oregano
- 1 teaspoon dried thyme
- 1 teaspoon fennel seeds
- 1 teaspoon freshly ground black pepper
- ½ teaspoon salt
- 1 cup mashed banana or applesauce

Directions:

1. Grease the insert of your Slow Cooker with olive oil
2. Take a large bowl and add pork, onion, banana/applesauce, almond flour, oregano, garlic, thyme, fennel seeds, pepper and salt
3. Mix well and pour the meat mix into the Slow Cooker
4. Shape it into loaf, leaving about ½ inch between the sides of the meat and inner pot wall
5. Cover and cook for 3 hours on LOW until the internal temperature reaches 150 degree Fahrenheit
6. Slice and serve
7. Enjoy!

Lunch recipes

Chicken and Celery Fries

Servings: 6

Prep +cook time: 35 minutes

Ingredients:Chicken

- Olive oil (2 T)
- Black pepper (.25 tsp.)
- Salt (.5 tsp.)
- Chicken breasts (4)

Ingredients:fries

- Black pepper (.25 tsp.)
- Salt (.5 tsp.)
- Olive oil (2 T)
- Celery (1.5 lbs.)

Directions:

1. Start by making sure your oven is heated to 400 degrees F.
2. Cut chicken into small pieces and place into a large mixing bowl before coating in oil and seasoning using spices. Let it marinate for a minimum of 15 minutes.
3. While the chicken marinates, cut the celery into strips before adding to a separate mixing bowl, coating in oil and seasoning with salt and pepper. Shake well.
4. Add the fries to a baking sheet and place them in the oven to bake 20 minutes.
5. Broil the chicken until its internal temperature reads at least 165 degrees Fahrenheit.

Sloppy Joe

Servings: 6

Prep +cook time: 75 minutes

Ingredients:

- Black pepper (as desired)Sea salt (as desired)
- Avocado oil (1 T)
- Pistachios (.25 c shelled)
- Water (.75 c)
- Chili (1 crushed)
- Paprika (.5 tsp.)
- Ginger (1 T minced)
- Garam masala (1 tsp.)
- Avocado oil (2 T)
- Garlic (1 clove minced)
- Avocado (1 mashed)
- Ground turkey (1 lb.)
- Avocado oil (2 T)
- White onion (.3 c diced fine)
- Cumin (1 tsp.)
- Apple cider vinegar (1 tsp.)
- Coconut milk (.25 c)
- Cilantro (1 handful chopped)

Directions:

1. Add 2 T avocado oil to a skillet before placing it on the stove over a burner turned to a medium/low heat and adding in the pistachios. Allow them to cook about 4 minutes and set aside.
2. Add 2 T avocado oil to a pot before placing in on a burner turned to a medium heat and adding in the ginger and garlic. Allow them to brown for 60 seconds before adding in the garam masala, water, mashed avocado, salt, paprika and chili. Allow the pot to simmer, covered while you complete the next steps.

3. Add the remaining avocado oil to the skillet before adding in the cumin and onions and stirring for 5 minutes before adding in the beef and the chilis. Brown the meat completely.

4. Add the skillet ingredients to the pot and turn up the heat to allow it to boil, removing the lid slightly to vent. Simmer for an additional 15 minutes on low/medium heat.

5. Add in the pistachios, vinegar and coconut milk and mix well prior to serving. Garnish with cilantro.

Ravioli and pesto

Servings: 1

Prep +cook time: 35 minutes

Ingredients:

- Parmesan cheese (.25 c)
- Mascarpone (.25 c)
- Coconut wraps (5)
- Eggs (2 beaten with 1 tsp. water)
- Coconut oil (4 T + .5 c divided)
- Frozen spinach (10 oz. thawed, dried)
- Pine nuts (.25 c)
- Garlic (2 cloves)
- Parmesan cheese (1 oz.)
- Basil leaves (2 c)
- Balsamic vinegar (as desired)
- Mixed salad greens (5 oz.)

Directions:

1. Ensure your oven is heated to 350 degrees F.
2. Add the coconut oil to a skillet before placing it on the stove over a burner turned to a medium heat. Add in the spinach and let it cook 2 minutes before removing it and placing it in a mixing bowl.
3. Add the .25 c parmesan cheese and the mascarpone to the bowl and mix well to combine thoroughly.
4. Line up 50 percent of the wraps on a cutting board before brushing them using the water and egg mixture. Place 1 T of the spinach mixture into each corner of each wrap, leaving as much space as possible between the scoops.
5. Brush one of the remaining wraps with the egg mixture and then use it to cover the tops of the filled wraps. Press down on the edges to create pockets and then use a ravioli cutter to cut out four squares total.
6. Add the remaining ingredients to a blender and blend well to create the pesto.

7. Place the rest of the coconut oil into a pan before placing the pan on the stove over a burner turned to a medium heat. Add the ravioli to the pan in batches, each should take about 2 minutes to cook, flip them at the 1 minute mark.

Bok choy and fried shrimp

Servings: 4

Prep +cook time: 10 minutes

Ingredients:

- Bok choy (.75 c)
- Garlic (.5 tsp.)
- Ginger (.25 tsp.)
- Sesame oil (.25 tsp.)
- Wild shrimp (24 oz.)

Directions:

1. Add all of the ingredients to a wok and stir fry for 10 minutes.
2. Serve hot.

Fettuccine

Servings: 4

Prep +cook time: 30 minutes

Ingredients:

- Black pepper (as desired)
- Sea salt (as desired)
- Mascarpone (1 c)
- Asparagus (1 bunch chopped)
- Parmesan cheese (.25 c grated)
- Shitake mushrooms (5 oz. sliced)
- Shirataki fettuccine noodles (32 oz. cooked)
- Extra-virgin olive oil (.25 c)
- Italian parsley (.5 c)
- Italian seasoning (.5 tsp.)

Directions:

1. Cook the pasta according to the provided instructions and keep 1 c of the water used to cook the noodles.
2. Add the oil to a skillet before placing it on the stove over a burner turned to a medium heat. Add in the mushrooms and increase the heat to high/medium and cook for 2 minutes before adding in the asparagus, the remaining oil and .5 tsp. salt. Cook until the asparagus is tender and crisp which should be about 3 minutes.
3. Turn off the heat before adding in the mascarpone and shirataki noodles before tossing to coat. Add .25 c of the reserved noodle water at a time to thin the sauce and keep the noodles moist. Stir in the remaining ingredients and serve warm.

Meatballs and salad

Servings: 6

Prep +cook time: 45 minutes

Ingredients:

- Black pepper (as desired)
- Sea salt (as desired)
- Raw honey (2 tsp.)
- Coconut aminos (1 T)
- Sesame coconut oil (1 T)
- Red pepper (.5 tsp.)
- Lime juice (3 T)
- Scallions (4 sliced thin)
- Cilantro (.5 c)
- Shitake mushrooms (.5 c sautéed)
- Meatballs (12 cooked)
- Baby bok choy (6 heads)
- Coconut oil (2 T)

Directions:

1. Add the coconut oil to a skillet before placing it on the stove over a burner turned to a medium heat. Add in the mushrooms and allow them to cook about 5 minutes. Add in the meatballs and let everything cook until they are warm.
2. In a serving bowl, add the honey, coconut aminos, sesame oil, red pepper and lime juice and mix well. Add in the scallions, cilantro, bok choy and the mixture from the skillet and toss to coat.

Chicken and cabbage with apples and cranberries

Servings: 4

Prep +cook time: 35 minutes

Ingredients:

- Black pepper (as desired)
- Sea salt (as desired)
- Apple cider vinegar (1 T)
- Ginger (1 tsp. ground)
- Chicken bone broth (.5 c)
- Apples (2 sliced)
- Chicken breast (2 lbs. boneless, skinless)
- Cranberries (1 c frozen)
- Raw honey (1 T)
- Cabbage (1 head cored)
- Cinnamon (1 tsp.)

Directions:

1. Add all of the ingredients to your Instant Pot and select the poultry setting prior to closing and securing the lid. Set the timer for 20 minutes.
2. Allow the pressure to release naturally for 10 minutes.
3. Serve hot and enjoy!

Mushroom mini pizza

Servings: 2

Prep +cook time: 35 minutes

Ingredients:

- Black pepper (as desired)
- Sea salt (as desired)
- Prosciutto (2 slices)
- Buffalo mozzarella (1 ball sliced)
- Basil pesto (6 T)
- Coconut oil (2 T)
- Portobello mushrooms (2 caps)

Directions:

- Ensure your oven is heated to 325 degrees F.
- Add the mushrooms caps to a baking pan before coating them in coconut oil. Place them in the oven for 5 minutes before removing the baking sheet from the oven, flipping the mushroom caps and returning them to the oven for an additional 5 minutes. The end result should be both crispy and brown on top.
- Add 3 T pesto to each cap, top with a slice of prosciutto and then the mozzarella.
- Return the mushrooms to the baking sheet and return the sheet to the oven for an additional 5 minutes.
- Season prior to serving hot.

Orange salmon salad

Servings: 4

Prep +cook time: 30 minutes

Ingredients:

- Black pepper (as desired)
- Sea salt (as desired)
- Dijon mustard (1 tsp.)
- Coconut oil (4 T)
- White wine vinegar (3 T)
- Raw honey (1 tsp.)
- Dill (1 T chopped)
- Lemon juice (1 lemon)
- Navel oranges (2 sectioned, peeled)
- Red onion (1 sliced thin)
- Salmon (1 lb. broiled, flaked)
- Baby spinach (5 oz.)
- Feta cheese (2 oz. crumbled)
- Hazelnuts (.3 c chopped, toasted)

Directions:

1. In a serving bowl, combine the flaked salmon, navel orange pieces, spinach and red onions.
2. In a separate bowl, add the feta cheese and hazelnuts and toss to combine before combining the two bowls and mixing well.
3. In a small bowl, mix together the Dijon mustard, coconut oil, white wine vinegar, honey, dill and lemon juice and whisk well.
4. Add the dressing to the salad and toss to coat.

Coconut chicken

Servings: 4

Prep +cook time: 30 minutes

Ingredients:

- Black pepper (as desired)
- Sea salt (as desired)
- Coconut milk (1 c)
- 5 spice powder (1 tsp.)
- Kosher salt (1 tsp.)
- Coconut aminos (3 T)
- Drumsticks (10 skin removed)
- Onion (1 sliced thin, peeled)
- Fish sauce (2 T)
- Ginger (1 in. peeled, chopped)
- Cilantro (.25 c)
- Garlic (4 cloves crushed, peeled)
- Lime juice (1 lime)
- Lemongrass (1 stalk chopped, skinned)
- Coconut oil (1 tsp.)

Directions:

- Add the ginger, fish sauce, garlic, lemongrass, coconut aminos and 5 spice powder in a blender before adding in the coconut milk and using the pulse setting to blend.
- Add the drumsticks to a bowl and season as desired before adding in the blender mixture and ensuring the drumsticks are well-coated.
- Turn on your Instant Pot and set it to the sauté setting and allow it to heat up before adding in the sliced onions and coconut oil and letting them cook about 5 minutes.
- Add the drumsticks and the marinade to the Instant Pot and select the warm option before sealing and locking the lid.
- Select the Manual option and then set the timer for 15 minutes and high pressure.
- Use the manual release valve when the drumsticks are done.

- Season with fish sauce prior to serving.

Arugula salad with sweet potato

Servings: 4

Prep +cook time: 20 minutes

Ingredients:

- Black pepper (as desired)
- Sea salt (as desired)
- Parmesan cheese (.25 c)
- Baby arugula (5 oz.)
- Dijon mustard (1 T)
- White wine vinegar (1 T)
- Swiss cheese (2 oz. shredded)
- Prosciutto (2 oz.)
- Sweet potat0 (1 lb. cubed, peeled)
- Coconut oil (.25 c)
- Tarragon leaves (.25 c chopped)

Directions:

1. Add your sweet potatoes to a boiler and then cover them with water. Allow them to boil before adding some salt and then reducing the temperature to let them simmer about 12 minutes. After they are done cooking drain them, run cold water oven them and then deposit them on a cutting board and dice them.
2. In a small bowl, combine the pepper, mustard, salt, oil and vinegar and mix well.
3. Split the arugula between 4 bowls before adding in the tarragon, sweet potatoes, prosciutto and swiss cheese. Top with dressing and parmesan prior to serving.

Enchiladas

Servings: 8

Prep +cook time: 45 minutes

Ingredients:

- Black pepper (as desired)
- Sea salt (as desired)
- Raw honey (1 tsp.)
- Paprika (.25 tsp.)
- Coconut aminos (1 tsp.)
- Oregano (.5 tsp. dried)
- Flour tortillas (8 warmed)
- Bone broth (2 c divided)
- Chicken (8 oz. shredded)
- Goat cheese (8 oz. crumbled)
- Cumin (.5 tsp. ground)
- Apple cider vinegar (3 tsp.)
- Garlic (4 cloves peeled)
- Shiitake mushrooms (8 oz. chopped)
- Olive oil (2 T)

Directions:

1. Ensure your oven is heated to 400 degrees F.
2. Add the oil to a skillet before placing it on the stove over a burner turned to a medium/high heat. Add in the mushrooms and onions and allow them to cook about 6 minutes, stirring regularly.
3. Mix in the pepper, salt and .5 c broth before reducing the heat to medium and letting everything cook about 4 minutes.
4. Once all the broth has been absorbed you will want to place all of the ingredients into a mixing bowl before stirring in half of the goat cheese.
5. Add the rest of the broth, paprika, oregano, honey, cumin, 2 tsp. sea salt, coconut aminos, garlic, apple cider vinegar and the rest of the broth in a blender and pulse until smooth. Add .5 c of the sauce to a glass dish (9 x 13).

6. Add .25 c of the mushroom mixture to each tortilla before folding up the bottom and then rolling it tightly. Place the finished tortillas into the baking dish and cover them with the sauce. Top all of the tortillas with the rest of the sauce and the remaining cheese.

7. Place the baking dish in the oven for about 15 minutes. You will know they are ready when the cheese is melted and the sauce is bubbling.

Baked sweet potato

Servings: 2

Prep +cook time: 20 minutes

Ingredients:

- Black pepper (as desired)
- Sea salt (as desired)
- Garlic (.25 tsp.)
- Kale (.5 c)
- Olive oil (.25 tsp.)
- Sweet potato (6 oz.)

Directions:

1. Ensure your oven is heated to 350 degrees F.
2. Add the sweet potatoes to pieces of aluminum foil, taking care to pierce the potato in numerous places to allow for venting. Coat the potatoes in the foil and then place them on a baking sheet.
3. Place the baking sheet in the oven and let them cook for 30 minutes, you will know they are ready wen they are soft all the way through.
4. Once they are finished cooking, remove the potatoes from the foil and place them in a large bowl. Mash the potatoes with the salt, pepper, garlic, olive oil and kale.

Celery soup

Servings: 4

Prep +cook time: 30 minutes

Ingredients:

- Black pepper (as desired)
- Sea salt (as desired)
- Coconut milk (1 c)
- Yellow onion (1 chopped)
- Water (2 c)
- Dill (.5 tsp.)
- Sea salt (1 pinch)
- Celery (1 bunch chopped)

Directions:

1. Add all of the ingredients to an Instant Pot and mix well. Seal the lid and choose the option for soup. This will warm the soup for 30 minutes before switching to a warming mode for a few hours.
2. Once the timer goes off select the option to manually vent the pressure.
3. Add the ingredients to an immersion blender and blend well.
4. Serve hot.

Sausage Risotto

Servings: 4

Prep +cook time: 30 minutes

Ingredients:

- Coconut oil (1 T)
- Summer squash (2 diced, seeded)
- Onions (2 c sliced)
- Cajun seasoning (1 T)
- Water (3.5 c)
- Leafy greens (2 handfuls chopped)
- Rope sausage (1.5 lbs. diagonally sliced)
- Arborio rice (2 c)
- Bell peppers (1.5 c diced)

Directions:

1. Add the spices and the salt to a small bowl and mix well before sprinkling over the top of the sausage and rubbing well.
2. Turn your pressure cooker to a high/medium heat and add in the coconut oil and allow it to melt before adding in the sausage and allowing it to cook about 3 minutes.
3. Add in the remaining ingredients and stir well before cooking an additional 3 minutes.
4. Sir in the remaining ingredients and close the lid before selecting the option for high heat and full pressure. Let everything cook for 5 minutes before letting it sit for 5 minutes and letting the pressure release an addition 3 minutes.
5. Add in the remaining seasoning and stir well prior to serving.

Dinner recipes

Spinach salad with steak

Servings: 4

Prep +cook time: 25 minutes

Ingredients:

- Black pepper (as desired)
- Sea salt (as desired)
- Red wine vinegar (2 T)
- Thyme (2 tsp. dried)
- Goat milk yogurt (4 oz.)
- Shirataki rice (1 c rinsed, drained)
- Baby spinach (5 oz.)
- Grass-fed steak (1 lb.)
- Pine nuts (2 T)

Directions:

1. Add the steak to a skillet before placing it on the stove over a burner turned to a medium heat. Prepare your steak to its desired level of doneness.
2. While the steak is cooking, add the pepper, salt, thyme, yogurt and red wine vinegar in a small bowl and whisk well.
3. Cook the rice according to instructions.
4. Plate the spinach in four separate bowls before topping with sliced steak, pine nuts, rice and dressing.

Squash soup

Servings: 4

Prep +cook time: 45 minutes

Ingredients:

- Black pepper (as desired)
- Sea salt (as desired)
- Thyme (2 T)
- Chives (2 T)
- Coconut milk (1 can)
- Oregano (2 T)
- Chicken stock (6 c)
- Garlic (4 cloves peeled)
- Celery (2 c)
- Salt (1.5 T)
- Herbs de Provence 93 T)
- Carrots (3)
- Cayenne pepper (.25 T)
- Onion (1 sliced)
- Butternut squash (1 peeled)
- Parsley leaves (.25 c)

Directions:

1. Slice the butternut squash in half before trimming off the ends and removing the seeds. Dice the remaining squash.
2. Add all of the ingredients, except the coconut milk to your pressure cooker, saving the chicken stock and seasonings for last.
3. Secure the lid of the pressure cooker and choose the soup option. Allow the Instant Pot to cook for 30 minutes and then release the pressure manually.
4. Pour the results into an immersion blender and blend your soup until smooth.
5. Add in the coconut milk and season as desired.
6. Serve hot.

Sweet potato gnocchi

Servings: 4

Prep +cook time: 60 minutes

Ingredients:

- Black pepper (as desired)
- Sea salt (as desired)
- Parmesan cheese (.25 c)
- Lemon (1 zested, juiced)
- Garlic (1 clove crushed)
- Coconut oil (3 T)
- Basil (.5 c torn, divided)
- Sweet potato (peeled, chunked)
- Egg (1)
- Sea salt (.5 tsp.)
- Cassava flour (.5 c)

Directions:

1. Place the sweet potatoes in a pot before filling the pot with water so the gnocchi is covered in about 2 inches of water before placing the pot on the stove over a burner turned to a high heat. Bring the pot to a boil before turning down the heat and allowing the pot to simmer for 15 minutes partially covered. Drain the potatoes, rinse them with cold water, and then drain.
2. Place the sweet potatoes in a bowl and mash them before adding in the egg and a pinch of salt. Add in the flour and the knead the mixture until it forms a dough. If the dough sticks to your fingers add more flour.
3. Add a pinch of salt to a pot of water before placing the pot on the stove over a burner turned to a high heat.
4. While waiting for the water to boil roll the dough into long, think rolls about the width of a thumb. Chop each roll into 1-inch pieces and put a shallow indent in each.
5. Place the gnocchi in the water using a slotted spoon. When they start to float they are ready to be removed. Place the finished gnocchi in a covered bowl to keep them warm.

6. Add the oil to the skillet before placing it on the stove over a burner turned to a medium heat. Add in the garlic and let it cook about 4 minutes before adding the gnocchi and basil to the skillet and mix well. Cook about 2 minutes before adding in the pepper, lemon zest, lemon juice and salt.
7. Top with cheese and basil prior to serving.

Chili

Servings: 8

Prep +cook time: 6 hours 15 minutes

Ingredients:

- Black pepper (as desired)
- Sea salt (as desired)
- Sweet potato puree (15 oz.)
- Red wine vinegar (2 tsp.)
- Chili powder (2 T)
- Celery (3 ribs diced fine)
- Onion (1 diced)
- Beef bone broth (2 c)
- Cloves (1 pinch ground)
- Cinnamon (1 pinch ground)
- Adobo sauce (1 T)
- Cumin (2 tsp. ground)
- Garlic (4 cloves minced)
- Grass-feed beef (2 lbs. ground)
- Avocado oil (1 T divided)
- Coconut aminos (2 tsp.)

Directions:

1. Add the coconut oil to a skillet before placing it on the stove over a burner turned to a high heat. Add in .5 tsp. salt along with the ground beef and allow the meat to brown, using a spatula to break it up as you go. After about 5 minutes place the meat in your slow cooker.
2. Reduce the burner heat to medium before adding in another tsp. of oil along with the onion, celery and garlic. Let everything cook for 5 minutes before adding in the chili powder, cinnamon, cloves and cumin. Let everything cook an additional 60 seconds while you stir. Add in the bone broth and let everything cook an additional 30 seconds before adding the contents of the skillet to the slow cooker.
3. Add in the coconut aminos, vinegar, adobo sauce, sweet potato puree and season as desired.

4. Cover the slow cooker and allow it to cook on a low heat for 6 hours.
5. Top with lime wedges, scallions and sour cream prior to serving.

Taco cups

Servings: 12

Prep +cook time: 90 minutes

Ingredients:

- Black pepper (as desired)
- Sea salt (as desired)
- Chili powder (2 tsp.)
- Black beans (2 cans)
- Garlic powder (.25 tsp.)
- Onion (1 chopped fine)
- Avocado oil (3 T)
- Paprika (.5 tsp.)
- Coriander (1 tsp.)
- Palm shortening (.25 c)
- Coconut milk (.5 c room temp.)
- Cassava flour (1 c)
- Coconut aminos (1 tsp)
- Oregano (.5 tsp. dried)
- Water (.25 c)
- Taco cups (12)
- Ground cumin (2 tsp.)

Directions:

1. Ensure your oven is heated to 425 degrees F.
2. Prepare a muffin pan by turning it upside down and greasing it using 1 T avocado oil.
3. In a mixing bowl, combine the water, palm shortening, cassava flour and coconut milk together and blend well.
4. Form the resulting dough into 12 single oz. balls before rolling each ball out flat and placing them between 2 pieces of parchment paper
5. Add the coconut oil to a skillet before placing it on the stove over a burner turned to a medium heat.

6. Place the pieces of dough over the underside of the muffin cups to create bowls. Place the muffin tin in the oven for 20 minutes.

7. Let the cups cool prior to filling.

8. While the cups are baking, add the remaining oil to a skilling before placing it on top of a burner turned a medium heat. Add in the onions and let them cook for 2 minutes, stirring constantly. Add in the spice and coconut aminos and ensure the onions are well-coated before letting them cook an additional 60 seconds while stirring.

9. Add the onions and black beans to the Instant Pot and season as desired. Close and seal the Instant Pot and turn it to a high pressure and cook 5 minutes. Let the pressure release naturally before seasoning as desired.

10. Fill taco cups prior to serving.

Stuffed peppers

Servings: 6

Prep +cook time: 6 hours 10 minutes

Ingredients:

- Thyme (2 tsp. dried)
- Oregano (2 tsp. dried)
- Basil (2 tsp. dried)
- Garlic (.5 clove minced)
- White onion (1 small, diced)
- Cauliflower (.5 head processed to resemble rice)
- Bell peppers (5 seeded, peeled)
- Italian hot sausage (1 lb.)

Directions:

1. Start by removing the top part of each pepper from the rest of the pepper. Save the top part of each pepper but remove and discard the seeds.
2. Add the processed cauliflower to a mixing bowl before mixing in the onion, garlic, basil, thyme and oregano and combining well.
3. Add the sausage to a skillet and place the skillet on the stove over a burner turned to a high/medium heat until it sears just enough to add to the favor.
4. Add the sausage to the bowl of cauliflower and mix well.
5. Add the results to the hollowed out peppers before placing each into your slow cooker and adding the tops of the peppers back in as well.
6. Cover the slow cooker and let it cook on a low heat for 6 hours.
7. Serve hot and enjoy.

Curry with Pineapple

Servings: 6

Prep +cook time: 6 hours 5 minutes

Ingredients:

- Black pepper (to taste)
- Salt (to taste)
- Lime juice (1 lime)
- Sweet potatoes (3 cups cubed)
- Carrot (3 chopped)
- Garlic (1 clove minced)
- Onion (.5 large diced)
- Garam masala (2 tsp.)
- Turmeric powder (.25 tsp.)
- Curry powder (.5 T)
- Vegetable stock (1 cup)
- Pumpkin puree (2 cups)
- Coconut milk (15 oz. unsweetened, full fat)

Directions:

1. Add the pepper, salt, Garam masala, turmeric powder, curry powder, vegetable stock, pumpkin puree and coconut milk to the slow cooker before mixing well.
2. Mix in the lime juice, sweet potatoes, carrots, garlic and onion and stir well.
3. Cover the slow cooker and let it cook on a low heat for 6 hours.
4. Serve hot over rice and enjoy.

Pot Roast

Servings: 6   **Prep +cook time: 7 hours 10 minutes**

Ingredients:

- Parsley (1 T chopped)
- Garlic (3 cloves chopped)
- Onion (.5 sliced)
- Celery (2 stalks diced)
- Carrots (5 diced, peeled)
- Beef stock (1 cup)
- Coconut oil (1 T)
- Beef roast (3 lbs. fat removed)
- Allspice (.5 tsp. ground)
- Clove (.5 tsp. ground)
- Salt (1.5 tsp. ground)
- Cinnamon (2 tsp.)
- Coriander (1 T ground)
- Pepper (1 T)

Directions:

1. Combine the allspice, clove, salt, cinnamon, coriander and pepper together and spread it over the meat.
2. Place a skillet on the stove over a burner with the heat turned to medium before adding the coconut oil.
3. Place the roast in the skillet and sear each side for a total of 10 minutes.
4. Place the roast in the slow cooker along with the celery, garlic, onion and carrots.
5. Add in the broth and let the slow cooker cook at a low temperature for 7 hours.
6. Add the parsley on top, serve and enjoy.

Salmon with Capers

Servings: 4

Prep +cook time: 30 minutes

Ingredients:

- Olive oil (to taste)
- Salt (to taste)
- Pepper (to taste)
- Thyme (1 T crushed)
- Capers (1 T)
- Lemon (1 thinly sliced)
- Salmon (32 oz.)

Directions:

1. Cover a baking sheet with a rim in parchment paper.
2. Put the salmon onto the baking sheet so that its skin touches the baking sheet.
3. Add salt and pepper to the fish as you prefer before topping the fish with the caper, thyme and lemon.
4. Place the fish in a cold oven, set the oven at 400 degrees Fahrenheit and let the fish cook for 25 minutes.
5. Serve hot and enjoy.

Squash and Thai Curry

Servings: 4

Prep +cook time: 30 minutes

Ingredients:

- Cauliflower rice (preparation details described below)
- Cilantro (.25 cups chopped)
- Lime juice (2 tsp.)
- Acorn Squash (1 peeled, seeded and cubed)
- Coconut aminos (1 T)
- Coconut milk (14 oz. can)
- Red curry paste (3 T)
- Ginger (1-inch peeled, minced)
- Garlic (4 cloves minced)
- Bell pepper (1 sliced)
- Salt (1 T)
- Onion (1 diced)
- Coconut oil (1 T)

Directions:

1. Place a large pan on a burner which has been turned to a medium heat.
2. Add in the coconut oil and the onion and let it cook for 6 minutes, be sure to stir.
3. Mix in the salt, ginger, garlic and bell pepper and let cook for 60 seconds.
4. Mix in the curry paste and let cook for an additional 60 seconds.
5. Mix in the coconut aminos and milk before bringing the pan to a simmer.
6. Mix in the squash and let the pan simmer for 20 minutes or until the squash has begun to grow tender.
7. Take the pan from the heat, mix in the lime juice.
8. Serve with cauliflower rice.

Chicken Pesto

Servings: 4

Prep +cook time: 45 minutes

Ingredients:

- Black pepper (as desired)
- Sea salt (as desired)
- Olive oil (4 T)
- Leafy greens (5.3 oz.)
- Garlic (1 clove chopped fine)
- Feta cheese (8 oz. diced)
- Olives (8 T pitted)
- Heavy whipping cream (1.5 c)
- Green pesto (3 oz.)
- Butter (2 oz.)
- Chicken thighs (1.5 lbs.)

Directions:

1. Ensure your oven is heated to 400F.
2. Cut the chicken into pieces before seasoning as desired and frying until it reaches an internal temperature of 165F.
3. In a small mixing bowl, combine the heavy cream and the pesto.
4. Add the chicken to a baking dish before adding in the garlic, feta cheese and olives and topping everything with the pesto mixture.
5. Place the dish in the oven and let it cook for 30 minutes.

Meat Pie

Servings: 4

Prep +cook time: 15 minutes

Ingredients:Filling

- Water (.5 c)
- Dried oregano (1 T)
- Sea salt (as desired)
- Black pepper (as desired)
- Ground lamb (1.3 lbs.)
- Olive oil (2 T)
- Garlic (1 clove chopped fine)
- Yellow onion (.5 chopped fine)

Ingredients:Crust

- Water (4 T)
- Egg (1 large, organic)
- Coconut oil (3 T)
- Salt (1 pinch)
- Baking powder (1 tsp.)
- Psyllium husk powder (1 T)
- Coconut powder (4 T)
- Almond flour (.75 c)

Ingredients:Toppings

- Shredded cheese (7 oz.)
- Cottage cheese (8 oz.)

Directions:

1. Ensure your oven is heated to 350F.
2. Add the olive oil to a skillet before placing it on the stove over a burned turned to a high/medium heat. Add in the garlic along with the onion and let them fry for 3 minutes or until they have softened.

3. Add in the ground beef, basil and oregano and season as desired before adding in the tomato paste as well as the water. Reduce the heat and let everything simmer 20 minutes. While this is taking place, make the crust.
4. Combine the dough ingredients using a food processor and process until the results form a ball. The same effect can be achieved by hand mixing with a fork.
5. Line greased 10-inch springform pan before spreading in the dough.
6. Bake the crust for 15 minutes before removing it and adding in the filling.
7. Mix together the shredded cheese and cottage cheese and add this on top.
8. Bake 30 minutes and let sit 5 minutes prior to baking.

Turkey Wings

Servings: 4

Prep +cook time: 30 minutes

Ingredients:

- Chopped thyme (1 bunch)
- Orange juice (1 c.)
- Chopped yellow onion (1)
- Pepper
- Salt
- Walnuts (1 c.)
- Dried cranberries (1.5 c.)
- Olive oil (2 Tbsp.)
- Coconut oil (2 T melted)
- Turkey wings (4)

Directions:

1. Set your Instant Pot on Sauté mode and add the oil and ghee. When these are warm, add the pepper, salt, and turkey wings. Let the wings heat up on all sides.
2. Add the thyme, cranberries, walnuts, and onion. Stir these around and cook for two minutes.
3. Add the orange juice and then cover up the pot. Cook these on High for 20 minutes.
4. Divide up the wings between a few plates and keep them warm.
5. Set the pot to Simmer mode and cook your cranberry mix for another 5 minutes. Drizzle this on the turkey wings and serve.

Meatballs

Servings: 3

Prep +cook time: 40 minutes

Ingredients:

- Coconut oil (2 T)
- Pepper (as desired)
- Salt (as desired)
- Oregano (1 T)
- White onion (2 T diced)
- Garlic (2 T minced)
- Bacon (9 slices)
- Italian sausage (1 lb.)

Directions:

- Start by making sure your oven is heated to 375F.
- Cover a baking sheet using aluminum foil.
- Place a skillet on top of a burner that has been turned to a high/medium heat before adding in the coconut oil and the sausage and letting it brown.
- Add all of the ingredients, save the bacon to a mixing bowl and combine thoroughly.
- Form the results into 9 meatballs and wrap a slice of bacon around each before placing them on the baking sheet. Place the baking sheet in the oven for 30 minutes or until the bacon is well-cooked.
- Let cool 5 minutes prior to serving.

Sliders

Servings: 6

Prep +cook time: 45 minutes

Ingredients:

- Water (.25 c)
- Heavy cream (.25 c)
- Salt (.5 tsp.)
- Garlic powder (.5 tsp.)
- Cheddar cheese (4 oz.)
- Butter (2 oz. unsalted)
- Carbquik (2 c)
- Hamburger (1 lb.)
- Cheddar cheese (6 slices)

Directions:

1. Start by making sure your oven is heated to 450F.
2. In a mixing bowl, add in the Carbquick before adding in the butter and mixing until the results start to form a dough.
3. Add in the garlic powder, cheese and salt and mix well before adding in the liquid ingredients and mixing to form a dough.
4. Form the dough into 6 equal sections and place them onto a prepared baking sheet.
5. Place the baking sheet in the oven for 8 minutes until the biscuits are golden brown.
6. While the biscuits are baking, place the hamburger into a skillet and place the skillet on top of a burner turned to a high/medium heat. As the meat browns, form it into small patties.
7. Slice the biscuits in half, and a hamburger patty and slice of cheese to each.

Burger with egg

Servings: 3

Prep +cook time: 30 minutes

Ingredients:

- Cheddar cheese (8 oz.)
- Worcestershire sauce (to taste)
- Onion powder (.5 tsp.)
- Garlic powder (.5 tsp.)
- Egg (2)
- Ground beef (1.5 lbs.)
- Coconut oil (2 T)
- Bacon (4 strips)

Directions:

1. In a mixing bowl, combine the eggs and beef and mix well before adding in the spices and combining thoroughly.
2. Break the results down into 1.5 oz. patties before topping each patty with .5 oz. of cheese.
3. Combine every 2 patties into a single burger.
4. Add the coconut oil to a pan before placing the pan on the stove on top of a burner turned to a high/medium heat. Add in one of the patties and cook each side for approximately 2 minutes or until it reaches your desired level of doneness.
5. In a separate frying pan, add in the bacon before placing it on top of a burner turned to a high/medium heat and cook until crispy.
6. Top each patty with bacon prior to serving.

Butternut and Chard Soup

Servings: 6

Prep +cook time: 20 minutes

Ingredients:

- Coconut cream (1 c.)
- Minced garlic cloves (4)
- Cubed butternut squash (2 c.)
- Hopped Swiss chard (4 c.)
- Chopped rosemary (1 tsp.)
- Pepper
- Salt
- Chicken stock (8 c.)
- Thyme sprigs (4)
- Chopped celery stalks (3)
- Chopped carrots (3)
- Chopped yellow onion (1)
- Olive oil (1 Tbsp.)

Directions:

1. Set the Instant Pot to Sauté mode before adding the oil. Add the celery, onion, and carrots.
2. After those are warm, add the rosemary, garlic, butternut squash, pepper, salt, chicken stock, and thyme. Stir and cook this on a high setting for 18 minutes.
3. Discard the thyme and add the coconut cream and Swiss chard. Warm up before serving.

Garlic Pot Roast

Servings: 8

Prep +cook time: 5 hours 10 minutes

Ingredients:

- Salt (as needed)
- Pepper (as needed)
- Beef stock (.75 cups)
- Garlic (1 tsp. minced0
- Bacon (6 slices, crumbled cooked)
- Beef shoulder (3 lbs.)

Directions:

1. Add the roast to the slow cooker and season as desired before topping with bacon and minced garlic.
2. Add in the beef stock and set the slow cooker, covered, to high and let everything sit for 5 hours until the meat has reached its desired level of tenderness.

Chicken and blackberry mustard

Servings: 4

Prep +cook time: 20 minutes

Ingredients:

- Blackberries (1 cup chopped)
- Mustard (1.5 T)
- Honey (2 tsp.)
- Chicken tenders (1 lb. halved)
- Salt (.5 tsp.)
- Black pepper (.25 tsp.)
- Cornmeal (3 T)
- Coconut oil (3 T)

Directions:

1. Season the chicken as desired before adding it to a bowl of the cornmeal and coating well.
2. Add the coconut oil to the skillet before adding the skillet to a burner turned to a high/medium heat.
3. After the oil has melted, lower the heat to medium and add in the chicken and let each side cook for about 4 minutes. The internal temperature should read 165 degrees Fahrenheit.
4. Remove the tenders from the stove and let them cool for a few minutes prior to serving.
5. Add the mustard, honey and berries together, max and mix well.
6. Serve with the chicken and enjoy.

Fish sandwich

Servings: 4

Prep +cook time: 20 minutes

Ingredients:

- Salmon fillet (1 lb. quartered)
- Cajun seasoning (2 tsp.)
- Avocado (1 pitted, peeled)
- Mayonnaise (2 T)
- White rolls (4)
- Arugula (1 cup)
- Red onion (.5 cups sliced thin)
- Coconut oil (2 T)

Directions:

1. Coat the grill in coconut oil before ensuring it is heated to a high heat.
2. Coat the fish using the seasoning before adding it to the grill and let it cook for approximately 3 minutes on each side.
3. Mash the avocado before mixing it with the mayonnaise and spreading on the rolls prior to serving.
4. Season as required, serve hot and enjoy.

Flap steak

Servings: 6

Prep +cook time: 4 hours 30 minutes

Ingredients:

- Black pepper (as needed)
- Salt (as needed)
- Coconut oil (2 T)
- Mango Salsa (as needed)
- Cumin (.5 tsp.)
- Coriander (.5 tsp.)
- Lime juice (1 T)
- White onion (.25 minced)
- Olive oil (.5 cups)
- Parsley (1 cup packed)
- Cilantro (1 cup packed)
- Flap steak (2 lbs. sliced thin)

Directions:

1. In a food processor, combine .5 tsp. salt, cumin, coriander, lime juice, white onion, olive oil, parsley and cilantro and process well.
2. Add the steak and half of the contents of a food processor to a resalable plastic bag before placing in the refrigerator to marinate for 4 hours.
3. Let the steak sit at room temperature for half an hour before heating your grill to a high heat and cooking the meat for approximately 2 minutes on each side.
4. Top with the remaining marinade prior to serving.

Chowder

Servings: 5

Prep +cook time: 55 minutes

Ingredients:

- Black pepper (as needed)
- Salt (as needed)
- Parsley (.25 cups chopped rough)
- Bay leaves (2)
- Chicken broth (6 cups)
- Thyme (1 tsp. dried)
- Oregano (1 tsp. dried)
- Smoked paprika (1 tsp.)
- Garlic powder (1 tsp.)
- Garlic (2 cloves chopped)
- Yellow onion (1 chopped)
- Celery (4 stalks diced)
- Carrots (2 diced, peeled)
- Shrimp (1 lb. deveined, peeled)
- Bacon (1.5 lbs.)
- Cauliflower (1 head florets, steamed, pureed)

Directions:

1. Place a Dutch oven on the stove on top of a burner turned to a medium heat. Add in the bacon and let it cook until it reaches the desired level of crispness. Remove the bacon from the oven and add in the shrimp before seasoning as needed and cooking each side for 2 minutes.
2. Add in the garlic, onion, celery and carrots and toss them in the bacon fat. After you can begin to see through the onion, mix in the salt, thyme, oregano, smoked paprika and garlic powder and stir for 60 seconds.
3. Mix in the bay leaves as well as the chicken broth and the cauliflower. Mix in half of the cooked bacon and let it cook for 15 minutes.
4. Take the bay leaves out of the mixture before adding in the parsley and pureeing everything in the Dutch Oven.

5. Add in the shrimp and heat completely.
6. Garnish with parsley, olive oil and bacon prior to serving.

Instant Pot chicken

Servings: 4

Prep +cook time: 50 minutes

Ingredients:

- Black pepper (as desired)
- Sea salt (as desired)
- Cilantro (.25 c)
- Ginger (1 in. chopped fine)
- Apple cider vinegar (2 T divided)
- Coconut aminos (.25 c + 1 T)
- Lime juice (1 lime)
- Garlic cloves (4)
- Salt (.5 tsp.)
- Raw honey (2 T)
- Mango (1 chunks)
- Green onion (1 sliced)
- Red onion (.5 chopped)
- Fish sauce (1 tsp)
- Chicken bone broth (.5 c)
- Chicken thighs (8 deboned)
- Cooking fat (1 T)

Directions:

1. Heat your Instant Pot by pressing the sauté button before adding in the fat and allowing it to melt.
2. Add in the chicken thighs with the skin facing down and allow it to cook for 3 minutes before flipping and allowing it to cook for 2 minutes more.
3. Remove the chicken from the Instant Pot before adding in the garlic, mango and onion and allow them to cook about 5 minutes.

4. Cancel the Instant Pot's sauté option before adding in the chicken, 1 T apple cider vinegar, honey, fish sauce, coconut aminos, chicken bone broth, lime juice, cilantro and ginger and mix well.

5. Put the lid on the Instant Pot and select the poultry setting before choosing the option for high pressure which will automatically set a timer for 15 minutes.

6. Manually release the pressure fully before removing the lid and removing the chicken from the Instant Pot.

7. Add in the remaining apple cider vinegar and coconut aminos, along with a pinch of salt and return the Instant Pot to the sauté setting to allow the sauce to reduce until it reaches your desired level of thickness.

8. Plate chicken and top with sauce and green onion prior to serving.

Cream soup

Servings: 4

Prep +cook time: 20 minutes

Ingredients:

- Black pepper (as desired)
- Sea salt (as desired)
- Broccoli (2 c florets)
- Garlic (2 cloves chopped, peeled)
- Coconut milk (500 mL)
- Coconut flour (.25 c)
- Bay leaf (1)
- Rutabaga (2 c)
- Basil (.5 tsp. dried)
- Raw honey (1 tsp.)
- White onion (1 c diced)
- Beef bone broth (2 c)
- Grass-fed beef (1 lb.)
- Plantain (2 c)
- Cinnamon (.5 tsp.)
- Water (6 c)
- Carrots (1 c)

Directions:

1. Add the water to your Instant Pot and use the sauté option to bring it to a boil before adding in your meat and letting it cook about 3 minutes.
2. Drain the water and return the meat to the pot before adding in the bone broth as well as the vegetables before seasoning it with the cinnamon, herbs, salt and pepper and mixing well.
3. Cover and seal the Instant Pot before setting it to 20 minutes.
4. Use the quick release valve when time has elapsed and remove the vegetables and meat when it is safe to do so.
5. Return the Instant Pot to the sauté setting before adding in the honey, coconut flour and coconut milk and mix well.

6. Add in the broccoli and allow it to simmer before removing the cinnamon and bay leaf once the broccoli has finished cooking.
7. Add all of the ingredients to a blender and blend well
8. Season prior to serving.

Noodles with broccoli and pesto

Servings: 4

Prep +cook time: 20 minutes

Ingredients:

- Black pepper (as desired)
- Sea salt (as desired)
- Broccoli florets (1 c)
- Olive oil (.25 tsp.)
- Basil pesto (.5 c)
- Miracle noodles (1 bag cooked)

Directions:

1. Add the coconut oil to a skillet before placing it on the stove over a burner turned to a medium heat. Add in the broccoli florets, pesto and noodles and let everything cook about 10 minutes, mixing regularly.
2. Season as desired prior to serving.

Dessert recipes

Lemon Meltaway Balls

Servings: 8

Prep +cook time: 10 minutes

Ingredients:

- 1 1/2 cups almond flour
- 1/4 cup organic lemon juice
- 1/4 cup organic coconut oil
- 1/4 cup organic erythritol syrup
- 1/3 cup organic coconut flour
- 1 tablespoon organic lemon zest
- 1/2 teaspoon organic pure vanilla extract
- 1-2 pinches Himalayan pink salt

Directions:

1. Add everything to a processor and pulse until it forms a smooth dough.
2. Make small balls out of this mixture place them on a baking sheet.
3. Refrigerate them for 15 minutes.
4. Roll the balls in coconut oil, then in coconut flakes and sugar.
5. Again, place them in a baking pan lined with wax paper.
6. Refrigerate them for 30 minutes.
7. Enjoy.

Moringa Ice Cream

Servings: 4

Prep +cook time: 10 minutes

Ingredients:

- Ice cream:
- 1 can organic full-fat coconut milk
- 1/4 - 1/2 cup organic granular sweetener
- teaspoons organic moringa powder
- 1 teaspoon organic baobab powder
- For the mix-in:
- 1/2 cup organic raw cacao nibs

Directions:

1. Put everything into the blender jug.
2. Blend them together until smooth.
3. Transfer the mixture to an ice maker and churn it as per machine's instructions.
4. Stir in the cacao nibs before freezing it.
5. Place the cacao ice cream in the freezer for 1 hour.
6. Serve.

Chocolate Turtles

Servings: 4

Prep +cook time: 10 minutes

Ingredients:

- For the caramel mixture:
- tablespoons organic almond butter
- 1 tablespoon organic coconut oil
- 1 pinch Himalayan pink salt
- 1 1/2 cups organic medjool dates (pitted)
- 2 tablespoons water (filtered/purified)

For the mix-in:

- 1 cup organic pecans (chopped)
- For the chocolate coating:
- 1 cup sugar-free mini-chocolate chips
- 1 tablespoon organic coconut oil

Directions:

1. Blend the caramel mixture in a blender jug
2. Fold in the pecans and mix them gently.
3. Pour caramel mixture over a baking sheet lined with a wax paper spoon by spoon.
4. Place them caramel bites in the refrigerator for 30 minutes.
5. Now melt the chocolate chips with coconut oil in a bowl by heating in a microwave for 3 minutes.
6. Dip the caramel bites in the chocolate to coat them well.
7. Return the bites to the refrigerator for 30 minutes.
8. Serve.

Vanilla Bean Ice Cream

Servings: 2

Prep +cook time: 10 minutes

Ingredients:

- cups full-fat organic coconut milk
- 1/2 cup organic granular swerve
- 2 teaspoons organic vanilla extract
- 1 teaspoon organic vanilla bean powder
- 1 pinch Himalayan pink salt

Directions:

1. Put everything into the blender jug.
2. Blend them together until smooth.
3. Transfer the mixture to an ice maker and churn it as per machine's instructions.
4. Place the vanilla ice cream in the freezer for 1 hour.
5. Serve.

Chocolate Fudge Tarts

Servings: 4

Prep +cook time: 10 minutes

Ingredients:

For the crust:

- 1 cup organic walnuts
- 1 cup organic medjool dates (pitted)
- 1 tablespoon organic coconut oil

For the filling:

- 1/2 cup organic coconut oil
- 1/4 cup organic raw cacao powder
- 1/2 cup organic date nectar
- 1/2 cup organic almond butter
- 1 pinch Himalayan pink salt

Directions:

1. Crush and grind all the ingredients for crust in a food processor.
2. Divide this mixture into a greased muffin tray.
3. Press the mixture firmly in the cups.
4. Refrigerate the crust for 15 minutes.
5. Meanwhile, blend the ingredients for filling.
6. Fill the crust with the filling.
7. Refrigerate for 30 minutes.
8. Serve

Simple Chocolate Mousse

Servings: 2

Prep +cook time: 10 minutes

Ingredients:

- 1 cup organic full-fat coconut milk
- 1 tablespoon organic raw cacao powder
- tablespoons organic unrefined granular sweetener

Directions:

1. Put everything into a blender jar.
2. Pulse the ingredients together until smooth.
3. Refrigerate well until chilled.
4. Serve with desired garnish.
5. Enjoy.

Pistachio Sesame Seed Balls

Servings: 6

Prep +cook time: 10 minutes

Ingredients:

- 1/2 cup organic almond butter
- 1/2 cup organic pistachios
- 1/2 cup organic sesame seeds
- 1 cup organic medjool dates (pitted)
- 1 tablespoon organic coconut oil

Directions:

1. Put everything into a food processor except sesame seeds.
2. Press the button to coarsely chop the mixture.
3. Fold in the sesame seeds and mix well with your hands.
4. Make small balls out of this mixture.
5. Refrigerate them for 30 minutes.
6. Serve and enjoy.

Pecan Pie Truffles

Servings: 4

Prep +cook time: 10 minutes

Ingredients:

- 1 cup organic pecans
- organic medjool dates (pitted)
- 1/2 teaspoon organic vanilla bean powder

Directions:

1. Coarsely grind every ingredienttogether in a food processor.
2. Make small balls out of the well-combined mixture.
3. Refrigerate for 15 minutes.
4. Serve and enjoy.

Snacks and Smoothies recipes

Mashed Cauliflower And Garlic

Servings: 4

Prep +cook time: 10 minutes

Ingredients:

- Ice cream:
- 1 can organic full-fat coconut milk
- 1/4 - 1/2 cup organic granular sweetener
- teaspoons organic moringa powder
- 1 teaspoon organic baobab powder
- For the mix-in:
- 1/2 cup organic raw cacao nibs

Directions:

1. Put everything into the blender jug.
2. Blend them together until smooth.
3. Transfer the mixture to an ice maker and churn it as per machine's instructions.
4. Stir in the cacao nibs before freezing it.
5. Place the cacao ice cream in the freezer for 1 hour.
6. Serve.

A Pot Full Of Pecans

Servings: 6

Prep +cook time: 3 hours 10 minutes

Ingredients

- 3 cups raw pecans
- ¼ cup date paste
- 2 teaspoons vanilla bean extract
- 1 teaspoon sea salt
- 1 tablespoon coconut oil

Directions

1. Add all of the listed ingredients to your pot
2. Cook on LOW for about 3 hours, making sure to stir it from time to time
3. One done, allow it to cool and serve!

Hot Buffalo Chicken Wings

Servings: 8

Prep +cook time: 6 hours 10 minutes

Ingredients

- 1 bottle of (12 ounce) hot pepper sauce
- ½ cup melted ghee
- 1 tablespoons dried oregano
- 2 teaspoons garlic powder
- 1 teaspoon onion powder
- 5 pounds chicken wing sections

Directions

1. Take a large bowl and mix hot sauce, ghee, garlic powder, oregano, onion powder and mix
2. Add chicken wings and toss them to coat well
3. Pour mix into Slow Cooker insert
4. Cover and cook on LOW for 6 hours
5. Serve and enjoy!

Hungry Dijon Potato

Servings: 4

Prep +cook time: 10 hours 15 minutes

Ingredients

- 1-2 tablespoons Dijon mustard
- 1 tablespoon olive oil
- 2 tablespoon apple cider vinegar
- Salt and pepper as needed
- 1 teaspoon dried rosemary
- 4 medium potato, peeled and cubed
- 11 medium onions, chopped

Directions

1. Take a medium sized bowl and add mustard, apple cider and oil
2. Mix them well and season the mixture with salt and pepper
3. Add potatoes and onion and give it a nice stir
4. Grease your slow cooker with cooking spray and transfer the prepared mixture to your Slow Cooker
5. Cover and cook on LOW for 10 hours
6. Once the potatoes are tender, enjoy!

Lovely Cashew Mix

Servings: 6

Prep +cook time: 2 hours 10 minutes

Ingredients

- 6 cups cashews
- 3 tablespoons coconut oil
- 1 tablespoon stevia
- Pinch of salt
- 2 tablespoon dried thyme
- 3 tablespoons dried rosemary leaves
- ¾ teaspoon paprika
- ½ teaspoon onion powder
- ½ teaspoon garlic powder

Directions

1. Heat your Slow Cooker by setting it to HIGH settings (for 15 minutes)
2. Add cashews and drizzle coconut oil over the cashews
3. Take a small bowl and add the spices, mix them well
4. Add the spices over the cashews and toss to coat them
5. Cover with lid and cook on LOW for 2 hours, making sure to keep stirring it after every hour
6. Remove the lid and cook for 30 minutes more
7. Serve and enjoy!

Lovely Potato Hash

Servings: 2

Prep +cook time: 4 hours 10 minutes

Ingredients:

- 1 medium orange pepper, sliced and diced, deseeded
- 1 medium yellow pepper, sliced and diced, deseeded
- 10 and ½ ounces sweet potato
- 1 tablespoon coconut oil
- 1 teaspoon garlic puree
- 1 teaspoon thyme
- 1 teaspoon mustard powder
- Salt and pepper as needed

Directions

1. Dice the vegetables and potatoes and transfer to your Slow Cooker
2. Add coconut oil and seasoning
3. Cover with lid and cook on LOW for 4 hours
4. Serve and enjoy!

Herbed Mushrooms

Servings: 4

Prep +cook time: 4 hours 20 minutes

Ingredients

- 24 ounce cremini mushrooms
- 4 garlic cloves, minced
- ½ teaspoon dried basil
- ½ teaspoon dried oregano
- 2 tablespoon parsley, minced
- 1 bay leaf
- 1 cup vegetable stock
- ¼ cup coconut milk
- 2 tablespoon ghee
- Sea salt as needed
- Freshly ground black pepper

Directions

1. Add the mushrooms, herbs and garlic to your slow cooker
2. Pour vegetable stock to the cooker and season
3. Cover and cook on LOW for 4 hours
4. Add coconut milk, stir and cook for a while until it is warm
5. Discard the bay leaf and season again
6. **Serve!**

Recipe index

Delicious Ginger Sweet Potatoes

Servings: 8

Prep +cook time: 4 hours 10 minutes

Ingredients

- 2 and ½ pound sweet potatoes, peeled
- 1 cup water
- 1 tablespoon fresh ginger, grated
- ½ teaspoon ginger, minced
- ½ tablespoon ghee

Directions

1. Peel the potatoes and quarter them
2. Add them to the slow cooker
3. Add water, fresh ginger and ginger
4. Stir well
5. Cook on HIGH for 3-4 hours until the potatoes are tender
6. Add ghee and mash them
7. Serve immediately and enjoy!

Caramelized Onion With Dope Garlic

Servings: 3

Prep +cook time: 10hours 20 minutes

Ingredients

- 10 large yellow onions, peeled and sliced
- 20 garlic cloves, peeled
- ¼ cup olive oil
- ¼ teaspoon salt
- 2 tablespoons balsamic vinegar
- 1 teaspoon dried thyme leaves

Directions

1. Add the listed ingredients to your Slow Cooker
2. Stir well
3. Cover and cook on LOW for 8-10 hours
4. Serve and enjoy!

Almond Fudge Cups

Servings: 6

Prep +cook time: 10 minutes

Ingredients:

For the fudge:

- 1 cup almonds, chopped
- 1 cup organic coconut oil, melted
- 1/4 cup raw cacao powder
- 1/4 cup date nectar
- 1/4 cup almond butter
- For the topping:
- sea salt

<u>Directions</u>:

1. Put everything for almond fudge cup in a bowl and mix them well.
2. Divide the mixture into 24 muffin cups.
3. Place the muffin cups in the refrigerator for 10 minutes.
4. Sprinkle sea salt on top of them.
5. Return them to the refrigerator for 1 hour.
6. Serve.

Herbal Fruit Stew

Servings: 8

Prep +cook time: 8 hours 10 minutes

Ingredients

- 2 cups dried apricot
- 2 cups prunes
- 2 cups pears
- 2 cups dried apples
- 1 cup dried cranberries
- 2 tablespoons stevia
- 6 cups water
- 1 teaspoon dried thyme leaves
- 1 teaspoon dried basil leaves

Directions:

1. Add the listed ingredients to your Slow Cooker
2. Cover and cook on LOW for 6-8 hours
3. Serve and enjoy!

Feisty Potato Grain

Servings: 8

Prep +cook time: 9 hours 10 minutes

Ingredients

- 6 Yukon Gold Potatoes, thinly sliced
- 3 sweet potatoes, thinly sliced and peeled
- 2 onions, thinly sliced
- 4 garlic cloves, minced
- 3 tablespoons almond flour
- 4 cups almond milk
- 1 and1/2 cups roasted veggie broth
- 3 tablespoons ghee
- 1 teaspoon dried thyme leaves
- 1 and ½ cup cashew cream

Directions

1. Grease your slow cooker with olive oil
2. Layer potatoes, onion and garlic
3. Take a large bowl and add flour, ½ cup milk and stir well
4. Stir in broth, ghee, thyme leaves
5. Pour milk mix over potatoes
6. Top with cashew cream
7. Cover and cook for 7-9 hours
8. Enjoy!

Conclusion

Just because you've finished this book doesn't mean there is nothing left to learn on the topic, expanding your horizons is the only way to find the mastery you seek.

When you are first making the transition to the lectin-free diet, it is important to always keep in mind that it isn't all or nothing. That is to say, just because you may find yourself in a situation where you aren't able to make a lectin-free choice, doesn't mean that you are somehow failing at the lectin-free diet. On the contrary, every single meal where you actively decrease the amount of lectin in your diet is a win and every meal where this doesn't happen is simply a chance to do better next time. As long as you don't let a single mistake turn into a prolonged binge of unhealthy foods full of lectin then there is nothing to hang your head about when you step out of line. Just remember, following the lectin-free diet is a marathon, not a sprint which means slow and steady will always win the race.